Innovation in Medical Technology

Innovation in Medical Technology

Ethical Issues and Challenges

MARGARET L. EATON

AND

DONALD KENNEDY

The Johns Hopkins University Press
Baltimore

© 2007 The Johns Hopkins University Press
All rights reserved. Published 2007
Printed in the United States of America on acid-free paper
2 4 6 8 9 7 5 3 1

The Johns Hopkins University Press
2715 North Charles Street
Baltimore, Maryland 21218-4363
www.press.jhu.edu

Library of Congress Cataloging-in-Publication Data
Eaton, Margaret L.
Innovation in medical technology : ethical issues and
challenges / Margaret L. Eaton and Donald Kennedy.
p. ; cm.
Includes bibliographical references and index.
ISBN-13: 978-0-8018-8526-6 (hardcover : alk. paper)
ISBN-10: 0-8018-8526-4 (hardcover : alk. paper)
1. Medical technology—Moral and ethical aspects.   2. Medical
innovations—Moral and ethical aspects.   3. Medical ethics.
I. Kennedy, Donald   II. Title.
[DNLM: 1. Technology Assessment, Biomedical—ethics.
2. Biomedical Research.   3. Diffusion of Innovation.
4. Professional Practice. W82 E14i 2007]
R855.3.E28 2007
174.2—dc22   2006019823

A catalog record for this book is available from the British Library.

Contents

Preface

Early in the current millennium, the Lasker Foundation[1] determined that it was time to examine the landscape of innovation in modern medical technology, to look at how new, unproved medical technologies are being deployed, and to identify ethical issues associated with this rapidly advancing arena of medical practice. This exploration began with a forum, the Lasker Forum on Ethical Challenges in Biomedical Research and Practice, held in Washington, D.C., at the American Association for the Advancement of Science on May 15 and 16, 2003. The forum was co-chaired by Drs. Donald Kennedy and Harold Shapiro,[2] assisted by the Planning Committee, whose names are listed in Appendix D. Attendance at the forum was by invitation only, and the attendees included some of the most influential thinkers in medicine, science, medical ethics, law, regulatory systems, and journalism, along with other stakeholders. The attendees are also listed in Appendix D. The Lasker Foundation principals and Drs. Kennedy and Shapiro were primarily interested in having this assembly investigate the adjoining areas of innovative clinical practice and more formal research. It was the committee's view that these two areas intersect to create a gray area, in which a given medical innovation can be considered either research (which must meet a variety of formal regulatory requirements) or innovative medical practice (which is governed by professional and malpractice standards). The objective of the forum was to map the modern terrain of this gray area by illuminating some ethical, legal, and social problem areas that lie within it.[3] The forum was designed to bring a multidisciplinary perspective to the topic and to consider the issues across medical specialties, each of which contributes a new dimension to the topic.

In preparation for the forum, participants were sent a series of hypothetical case studies and questions (all incorporated into this book); they were asked to come to the forum ready for debate and discussion. Over two days of intensive, directed discussions, the participants explored the question of how modern medical technology is naturally evolving and how that course can be better understood and perhaps improved. Using the case studies as the context in which to explore the issues, the participants wrestled with the ethical ramifications of various pathways of innovation. The authors of this book monitored the discussions and benefited from the notes taken by rapporteurs assigned to each case study section. We have included, in the discussion section of this book, much of what was learned from the process by which the forum was conducted. The statements made in this volume should not be taken as reflecting a consensus position of the participants in any session of the forum; often, there wasn't one. Nor have we used direct statements by individual participants. In a sense, this work consists of distillates from these rich and often lively sessions—supplemented by our own thoughts and the comments of others who have written on this topic. We hope we have captured some thoughtful and well-considered views from some of the country's best minds—people who spent considerable uninterrupted time focused on complex and important questions. This book is therefore the authors' effort to reproduce the work and thought that went into addressing medical innovation by the Lasker Foundation; Drs. Kennedy, Shapiro, and Eaton; the Lasker Forum Planning Committee; and the participants. The content and discussions were well received by those involved, and we hope that they will be enlightening and educational for others interested in this important subject.

The fundamental charge of the Lasker Forum participants was to focus on the overarching question of whether research or medical practice settings better serve medical innovation. In general, the participants wanted to be convinced that a particular new technology posed unacceptable risks before they would recommend deployment under a formal research protocol. Many participants believed that there were problems in each of the four medical practice areas discussed (off-label drug use, surgery, assisted reproduction, and neuroimaging) but that these problems did not rise to a level that would require all innovative medical technologies to be researched before offering them as patient care. Nor was such an approach considered feasible; instead, the assembly chose to focus on whether the process of medical innovation could be improved in less formal ways, namely, with nongovernmental oversight for some technologies, with better disclosure of information to patients for all technologies, and with better collection and publication of outcome data while innovation is ongoing.

The choice to address these three areas was made by the forum participants themselves—which raises the issue of the implications of that choice. Based on the discussions that took place, the first implication is that oversight, disclosure, and the duties to learn and educate are important considerations that should always be considered when deploying new medical technologies. Oversight is important to prevent scientific enthusiasm from leading to uncritical acceptance and a limited view of the wider consequences of medical innovation. It is equally important to ensure that oversight does not unduly inhibit innovation. Using significant risk as the measure with which to identify those technologies that need oversight addresses this concern. Disclosure focuses on the patient—the ultimate beneficiary and sometimes the unfortunate victim—of medical technology. Any attempt to weigh the ethical aspects of medical innovation must give primary interest to patient rights and must ensure that the imperatives of medical progress and social benefit do not trump these rights. The duties to learn and educate ensure that the information and the lessons, both good and bad, are captured and disseminated. Learning and educating promotes progress, and can prevent the harm to patients caused when a lack of outside scrutiny perpetuates the use of ineffective or unsafe medical technology.

The second implication of the Lasker Forum participants' three core concerns is that the lack of consensus in the medical profession regarding what are appropriate levels of oversight, patient consent, and sharing of information must be addressed. There was a wide range of opinion among participants about what standards should be met in these three areas, who should set the standards, and how each area should be managed. What constitutes appropriate technology oversight is a perennially debated topic among medical practitioners, policy makers, and in society generally. There is no agreement on which aspects of medical innovation should be left to the discretion of the profession (presumably the aspects that it knows and manages best) and which require extramural oversight. Also, accepting the primacy of patient autonomy has led to ongoing debates about what constitutes an informed and free choice to accept or reject new medical treatment (the risks and benefits of which may be technical and opaque to both the practitioner and the patient). And, while there was general agreement that learning from and disseminating information about medical innovations are worthy goals, no agreement exists about how to accomplish them. The range of opinions on these topics indicates that one product of further exploration of the landscape of innovation should be the development of standards or best practices in these three areas.

The goal, after all, is for advances in medical technology to optimally serve the interests of science, medical practice, patients, and society. Success will depend first on understanding how medical innovations are being deployed and on identifying the issues that arise from how that is done. The Lasker Foundation has made an effort to contribute to these first steps, and hopes that this text will enrich continuing education on this topic, one that is so important to the role of medicine in society and to our collective future health.

THE SCOPE OF THE BOOK

This book is written for those interested in studying the ethical, legal, and so-cial policy aspects of biomedical science, medical practice, and their regulation. Although not a prerequisite, users of the book will derive the most benefit if they have some basic familiarity with the guidelines, regulations, and laws that gov-ern medical research and medical practice. This background information will allow a fuller understanding of the consequences of choosing to innovate in med-icine under a research protocol or in a medical practice setting. For those who lack knowledge of the regulations or who are not familiar with medical tech-nologies, we have identified the regulations, defined terms, and described tech-nologies as much as was feasible without interrupting the discussion. The com-bination of background material, cases, and discussion is intended to supply information about the ways in which medical innovation takes place and, using the cases in particular, to stimulate reflection about and discussion of the re-sponsibilities attendant upon those who engage in and oversee this activity and of the broader issues associated with medical innovation.

CASE STUDIES

The case studies in this book deal with four types of unregulated or lightly reg-ulated medical innovation: off-label drug use, innovative surgery, assisted repro-duction, and neuroimaging. Case studies were used because it is much easier and more effective, in our opinion, to convey the complexities of medical innovation using realistic examples of how these processes evolve. The case studies are hy-pothetical and set in the near future but are based on an amalgam of real events that have occurred with past medical innovations. The technologies described in each case are extensions of existing medical practice and involve some procedures or methods that are not now in use but can realistically be expected to be forth-coming. (By the time this book is published and read, some of the anticipated technological advances are likely to have come into use.) Each case study is pre-ceded by background material discussing the technology and how it evolved. This material informs and illustrates many of the issues raised in each case. Questions follow each case to focus thought; they can also be used in an academic or policy-setting arena to direct discussion or to make the participants "work" to arrive at justifiable conclusions about how the innovative process should be handled.

THEMES FOR DISCUSSION

As at the Lasker Forum, the objective in discussing the cases and questions is to shed light on and respond to the many aspects of this issue. The Lasker Forum participants identified five themes as common to the leading edge of medical technology. These themes impinge on a central choice that must be made for any medical technological innovation.

The *central theme* is whether to deploy a new medical technology in the unregulated (or lightly regulated) clinical practice environment or in the research environment and thus within its regulatory regime. This choice raises many ethical dilemmas that affect patients, medical practitioners, the medical profession, and society at large. These ethical dilemmas can inspire questions such as:

- What principles govern the responsible introduction of innovative medical products and services into humans? The values associated with this question relate to scientific integrity and the obligations of medical science.
- What are the boundaries of the duty to protect patients from harm? The values associated with this question relate to paternalism and nonmalfeasance (doing no harm).
- How is meaningful patient consent assured? The values associated with this question relate to respecting and facilitating patients' liberty and autonomy.
- How is it assured that new therapies provide benefit to patients? The value associated with this question relates to beneficence (doing the good that one can).
- How are conflicts of interest to be managed or avoided? The value associated with this question relates to loyalty.
- What is the extent of the duty to mitigate harm? The value associated with this question relates to compensatory justice.
- Is there a duty to assure access to new medical therapies? The value associated with this question relates to distributive justice.

From these ethical issues, several *subthemes* can be explored:

Oversight. In an unregulated environment, it is often unclear whether a new technology should be subject to research controls or can be deployed as an innovative practice, where patients may have quicker access to therapies but the extent and quality of oversight may be ad hoc.

Impacts on Medical Science and Practice. When new medical technologies are deployed as innovative practice, preclinical testing and patient selection vary among practitioners and data gathering may be informal. As a result, there may be greater uncertainty about whether the procedures or materials are ready to be introduced into general practice. Another result is that valuable experiences and outcomes may not be made known to other members of the profession.

Patients' Concerns. Whether medical technologies are deployed as innovative practice or as regulated research, patients' interests and well-being should be balanced with the interests of promoting scientific and medical advances. Bearing on the concerns for patients' well-being are: anticipating and addressing both near- and long-term consequences for patients, protecting patients from harm, maximizing patient benefit, providing patients with information sufficient to allow them to understand the full consequences of a choice to accept or reject the intervention, protecting patients from coercion to accept the intervention, refraining from exploiting patient vulnerabilities, and safeguarding medical privacy.

Conflicts of Interests. Advanced medical technologies are frequently introduced in settings where several realms intersect—academic, medical practice, and commercial. This may create perceived or actual conflicts of interest, primarily financial or reputational.

Legal Consequences. Injuries experienced as a result of having been treated with innovative therapies will often be litigated, requiring courts to struggle with how to apply the law to novel claims and circumstances.

Our ultimate goal in presenting this information is to provide educational material about the nature and consequences of medical innovation and to contribute to the national discourse about how the value of modern technological development in medicine can best be preserved.

Acknowledgments

As described above, this book grew out of the Forum on Ethical Challenges in Biomedical Research and Practice, initiated and sponsored by the Albert and Mary Lasker Foundation with additional and very welcome support from the Walter and Elise Haas Fund, the Robert Wood Johnson Foundation, the Greenwall Foundation, and the American Association for the Advancement of Science. Together, these nonprofit organizations contributed generously to the exploration of a topic of vital interest to medical, patient, and policy communities.

Neen Hunt, the president of the Lasker Foundation, deserves special credit for envisioning the forum and shepherding it to completion. Thanks are owed also to the co-chair of the forum, Harold Shapiro, who was generous with his time, insights, and wisdom. Ticien Sassoubre was a terrific editor. Marty Krasny, the forum's coordinator, provided valuable guidance and advice. Anne Whitmore, at the Johns Hopkins University Press, was exceptional in copyediting the manuscript and managing the publication process. Finally, we thank all of those who attended the forum; their thoughtful insights and comments form the basis for the discussion contained in this book.

Innovation in Medical Technology

The Need to Ask Questions about Innovation

ready, resourceful man!
Never without resources
never an impasse as he marches on the future—
only Death, from Death alone he will find no rescue
but from desperate plagues he has plotted his escape

Man the master, ingenious past all measure
past all dreams, the skills within his grasp—
he forges on, now to destruction
now again to greatness. When he weaves in
the laws of the land, and the justice of the gods
that binds his oaths together
he and his city rise high—
but the city casts out
that man who weds himself to inhumanity
thanks to reckless daring.

—Sophocles, *Antigone* (442 B.C.E.)

What is admirable about human abilities? Should limits be placed on human ability and action? How does a daring person get into trouble? Constantly and confidently innovating with the goal of conquering disease and injury is one of mankind's most admirable activities. Limiting this endeavor should perhaps be considered only when the harms of medical innovation outweigh the benefits. Recognizing in advance when harms are likely to predominate is never easy, but, as Sophocles suggests, it may help to consider the "laws of the land" and the "justice of the gods"—in other words, to acknowledge the social contracts and moral responsibilities that temper "reckless daring."

Exploring these wider implications of the way in which modern pioneering medical technologies are introduced in the real world is the purpose of this book. The choice of conduit for introducing medical advances—as research or as a new way to practice medicine—generates the fundamental ethical and social policy issues in this domain. Many other issues and conflicts flow from this choice, especially because the pace, sophistication, and power of medical technology innovation have been rapidly increasing. Yet, few recent or comprehensive efforts have been made to address the ethical and social issues associated with this steady advance.

Medical innovation is perhaps best exemplified by the following circumstance. A skillful physician-scientist encounters a patient with an unexpectedly challenging life-threatening condition. Treatments meeting the usual medical "standard of care" have proved unavailing, but the physician—possibly encouraged by the results of animal experiments conducted in his laboratory—believes that a different kind of intervention could work. The novel treatment or procedure is applied, and the patient improves! Most practitioners and patients would applaud the physician for going forward—at least the first time. The level and persistence of approval might depend, of course, on just how far from standard the new intervention was and whether the physician intended to try the same thing again.

In the interest of patients in general, most practitioners and most medical organizations (professional societies, hospital boards, and the like) support innovative medicine that preserves health and saves lives. At some point, however, the decision must be made as to whether an innovation is to be regarded as a practice variation, lying clearly within the scope of the physician's initiative, or as something else. The "something else" would be research: clinical innovation conducted under a planned protocol, with its outcome carefully recorded, the process subject to a highly evolved system of oversight and rules designed to protect patients (read: human subjects) from the adverse consequences of premature use of a technology, of less than fully informed consent, and of overly enthusiastic recruitment.[1] Thus it is that innovation sometimes proceeds and spreads with little oversight, whereas at other times it is called research and made subject to extensive controls. That constitutes something of a paradox. Regulated research on humans is defined as: a systematic investigation designed to develop or contribute to generalizable knowledge (*Code of Federal Regulations*). If an innovating physician is not using systematic methods or intending to advance general medical knowledge, the innovative activity is not subject to regulatory control and supervision. That has led one observing ethicist to wonder why it is that "we regulate only when we expect to learn something!" That charge is not entirely fair, because there is an intermediate condition: although healing a sick patient may be the primary motivation of physicians applying new treatment methods, they often use an orderly approach, carefully record conditions and results, and publish the results of their innovative techniques. That kind of overlap between these two activities has created a gray area, in which some new medical treatments are deployed in an arena that has intentional and outcome aspects of both research and medical practice.

This gray area constitutes the main focus of this book. We deal here with medical technologies and therapies that are created and exist outside of regulatory jurisdiction where the physician can choose how to innovate. Our exploration of this terrain is from the viewpoint of the physician who decides to innovate and to advance patient care without the benefits (or burdens) of research. We then address the consequences of that choice. In the process, we pose questions such as these: What path to innovation best advances patients' interests? Without careful research controls, how can the medical community know whether a particular innovation has real value? Do the requirements of research and regulation stifle medical progress? Do innovative physicians tend to take unreasonable risks on behalf of their patients? Without the regulatory controls, are physicians tempted to exclude the patient in making treatment choices?

Two articles published in the New Yorker fortuitously provide intellectual bookends for the discussion of medical innovation. Both were written by physicians who are also superb writers. The first, by Atul Gawande (Gawande 2003), was a long biographical sketch of an influential Harvard physician, Francis Moore, who was launched into a remarkable surgical career by his experience (as a young resident) in treating the burn victims of the famous 1942 Coconut Grove fire. The second, by Jerome Groopman (Groopman 2003), was built around long interviews with the actor Christopher Reeve, who, as nearly everyone now knows, was paralyzed by a cervical dislocation caused by an accident during an equestrian competition. The interplay between medical aggressiveness and risk, on the one hand, and caution and patient protection, on the other, forms a dramatic focus in both of these stories.

The young Dr. Moore (popular, and widely known around Harvard in those days as "Franny" Moore) was about as medically venturesome as it gets. He became the chairman of surgery at Harvard's Peter Bent Brigham Hospital at age 34, and he made a series of extraordinary research discoveries. As a clinician, he could be counted on to deploy and then advocate procedures that went beyond the "standard of care" boundary; and he became, at least around Boston, a kind of emblem for aggressive practice. Some of Moore's patients' lives were saved with dramatic new procedures that later became widely adopted. Other patients died during Moore's attempts to save them—risks Moore was willing to take in what he believed to be their best interest. But later in his career, after a series of spectacularly failed liver transplants, Moore had a conversion and never again experimented with a major new surgery on human beings. Instead, he became an advocate for perfecting all new procedures on animals before applying them in the care of human patients, and he wrote a series of studies evaluating the outcomes of innovative surgical procedures.[2] In the midarc of his career, Moore transformed himself from an aggressive young surgeon into a cautious elder who promoted rigorously evaluating new procedures before adopting them in practice. At the end of his account, Gawande—himself a young surgeon—asks himself which Moore he prefers—and inclines toward the young Moore.

Groopman's account of Reeve's effort is also dramatic. The actor, equipped with high intelligence, a powerful personality, and a huge incentive to get better, made an additional career of persuading scientists and doctors to get on with it. He was dissatisfied with the cautious, conventional medical wisdom about the improbability of neural regeneration and was impatient whenever he encountered any unwillingness to try new methods. Reeve told Groopman that he did not want reckless physicians, but neither did he want fearful ones. At some medical meetings, he annoyed his audiences by criticizing medical caution and pushing researchers to do more. One could say, of course, that Reeve's functional impairment, in addition to providing an incentive for cure, encouraged him to be overly tolerant of risk. Given the choice, it is fairly plain that he too would have preferred the young Franny Moore. How the author, as a physician, would have voted is much less clear.

To begin the exploration of our topic, it may be helpful to lay out the process by which innovative medical treatments and procedures evolve into accepted and established medical practice. Many new treatment modalities take a path well known to clinical scientists that involves a formal set of research procedures. A medical scientist adopts a hypothesis, perhaps on the basis of suggestive preliminary evidence, that a certain treatment or procedure will be safe and effective. He or she then tests that hypothesis in animal and then in human (i.e., clinical) research.

If the new treatment involves an FDA-regulated drug, device, or biological agent, the process of development is linear: it begins with laboratory studies, then moves through further animal tests, and then into three phases of human testing. In Phase I tests, increasing doses of the drug are given to healthy human subjects to establish safe levels. Phase II trials are often done in subjects with the disease for which the treatment is intended; typically these tests involve carefully selected patients in academic health centers, divided into matched groups that are randomly assigned to receive either the treatment or a look-alike placebo. These trials are often "double blind" in that neither the subject patients nor the physicians examining the health of the patients know which intervention the subjects received.[3] Phase III trials resemble those of Phase II but are usually larger in scale and involve patients in a variety of health care settings, to imitate the diverse conditions under which the new therapy may be employed. This entire process can take up to ten years and an expenditure of more than $800 million before drugs and biologics achieve FDA approval. Data showing that a treatment is safe and effective in such randomized, double-blind clinical studies are the most scientifically and medically persuasive; and if the process results in FDA approval, adoption of the treatment is often widespread.

Data from controlled studies falling short of this ideal, especially if they are published in a respected clinical journal, can spur treatment adoption, though to a lesser extent. Establishment of the value of a treatment in the medical armamentarium by carefully controlled research can occur at the beginning of innovation or after the treatment is already in widespread use, or anytime in between.

Because research of this kind involves human participants who are being subjected to as-yet-unproven therapies, a whole set of regulatory protections has been applied to it—institutional review boards (IRBs) and informed consent requirements among them.

A good example of how the other path to innovation begins is the following account:

> On the morning of August 16, 1985, Guy Condelli, a five-year-old boy who lived in the Boston suburb of Medford, Massachusetts, had his right ear bitten off by a dog. During a twelve-hour operation, Joseph Upton, a reconstructive plastic surgeon at Children's Hospital Boston and a professor at Harvard Medical School, reattached Condelli's ear. Three days later, however, it turned blue-black from venous congestion. The boy was given blood thinners and his ear was lanced, but the organ was dying. Upton had once read an article about the use of leeches to drain congested tissue and, desperate, decided to track some down.
>
> Upton had always been an adventurous doctor. As an Army surgeon during the Vietnam War, he had been posted at a large hospital in Augusta, Georgia, where

soldiers wounded in Southeast Asia were flown for treatment. Many arrived with infections. Upton knew that Civil War battlefield doctors had used maggots to remove infected tissue from wounds. (Maggots feed on necrotic flesh, leaving healthy tissue untouched.) He tried the technique and got splendid results. But when the Army hospital's chief of professional services realized what Upton was doing, he was threatened with a court-martial. With this experience in mind, Upton refrained from telling his superiors at Children's Hospital Boston about his plan to leech Condelli's ear. "If I had asked around Harvard—are you kidding me?" he says. Eventually, he reached Biopharm [a Welsh start-up company that supplied leeches for research and, in a small number of cases, for medical practice] and spoke to [the founder's wife], who drove a consignment of thirty leeches three hours from Swansea to London's Heathrow Airport and put them on a plane to Boston.

Upton attached two of the leeches to the upper helix of Condelli's ear, where the congestion was greatest. Within minutes, the organ began to turn pink, and after a few days it completely recovered. Upton became the first doctor to perform a successful microsurgical reattachment of a child's ear. The story became national news, and Upton began to get calls in the middle of the night from colleagues around the world asking, "Where do we get the leeches?" (Colapinto 2005, p. 77)

This example contains representations of most elements in the beginning phase of medical practice innovation. A physician is faced with a patient for whom existing treatment options have failed or, perhaps in a more usual scenario, sees a better way of combating a problem than the prevailing standard. The physician attempts a new approach and the patient improves. Or perhaps the patient fails to improve, but the physician thinks he or she knows why and can correct the failure. In either case, the treatment diffusion process usually begins when the physician believes that the treatment is worthwhile, uses it with increasing numbers of patients, and gets good results. The treatment may be inherently safe and effective, but in some cases, the enthusiasm with which the physician recommends the treatment can provoke a strong placebo effect in the patient, increasing the prospect for a spontaneous remission or other favorable response. It may also be that, unbeknownst to the physician, the patients are getting better spontaneously rather than as a result of the new treatment. Whatever the cause of the good results, the next step in the diffusion process occurs as the physician discloses the results to other practitioners, for instance during discussions at a professional conference. Word-of-mouth adoption is faster when innovations occur at an academic medical center, as is often the case. Students trained in the new techniques become a source of dissemination once they leave their training.

Dissemination happens even faster when the physician publishes a "promising report" in the medical literature (McKinlay 1981).[4] Many journals publish case reports of successful interventions used in one patient or a small number of patients. What can be learned from such reports? Unfortunately, physicians seldom learn from the mistakes or failures of their colleagues because negative case reports are not often published. And, although it is tempting to think that reports of successful outcomes mean that the intervention will work with other patients, few anecdotal reports control for the possibility that the good outcome was the result of some other factor. Nevertheless, case reports can prompt other physicians to adopt the practice, hoping for the same result. Adoption depends on many factors: how dire the medical condition was; how quickly and how well the intervention worked; how long the patients were followed; whether there are other treatment options; how many patients present with the same problem; how well known and respected the reporting physician is; how easily the innovation can be implemented; and whether the intervention will improve the potentially adopting physician's practice financially. Sometimes, the case report is followed by another, citing similar successes with a larger group of patients. These expanded reports are more persuasive and have a greater potential to change medical practice, despite still being considered anecdotal by most in the research community.

Another way word gets out about innovations is the pilot study, undertaken when a physician intends to develop a new therapy or procedure under a research protocol but needs preliminary information to properly design the study. The pilot study can provide information about the dosage of a drug or vaccine, the duration of follow-up needed to evaluate effects of the treatment, and the kinds of patient who should be excluded from the study. If the pilot study provides information needed to improve the ability to perform the research, all is well. Sometimes, the experience of the pilot study is so positive regarding safety and efficacy that the physician refrains from performing a formal study because it would deny the treatment to the subjects in the control group. In a few cases, new therapies were so remarkably effective in their early, nonformal trials that rigorous clinical trials seemed superfluous; among those are penicillin for pneumococcal infection, insulin for diabetes, and vitamin B_{12} for pernicious anemia. Highly effective treatment innovations such as these may thus become adopted on the evidence of a pilot study alone, especially if it is published.

Innovation may spread still faster when a promising report or controlled study is covered in the mass media as a "medical breakthrough." Increasingly, newspapers and magazines have been monitoring the medical journals to report on medical advances. Interviews with the innovating physician often result in highly optimistic quotes about the promise of the new treatment. Such reports can drive patients to their physician's office with demands for the treatment long before it has been validated by experience or research. For example, in 1998, Gina Kolata of the *New York Times* wrote a front-page article on the anticancer effects of two antiangiogenesis compounds called angiostatin and endostatin. These compounds had been discovered by Dr. Judah Folkman and were undergoing studies sponsored by Entremed, a biotechnology company. One promising study of Folkman's, performed on mice only, showed that these compounds not only stopped the spread of cancer but also eliminated existing tumors. Based on these findings, human trials were in preparation. In her article, Kolata quoted eminent scientists as saying, in effect, that the compounds were the single most exciting cancer treatment on the horizon (one even predicted that they would cure cancer in two years) and that they were being given top priority by the National Cancer Institute. As a result of the article, Entremed stock soared, television news reports of a "new cancer cure" appeared, and U.S. cancer clinics were swamped with phone calls from desperate patients seeking access to the two new "drugs." Some cancer patients even called their clinics saying that they wanted to delay starting chemotherapy until the new drugs were available (Cohen 1999; Shaw 2000). Had it been legal to prescribe those compounds for patients at that point, there undoubtedly would have been very strong pressure to do so.

Another stage in the process of dissemination occurs when the innovation is adopted or endorsed by a professional medical organization or hospital as safe and effective. Obviously, endorsement can be the result of the organization's belief that the innovation improves medical care. However, on occasion, other factors can influence adoption or endorsement decisions. These include peer pressure within the organization, the desire to maintain a reputation for being up-to-date or advanced, pressure from patient groups, or the influence of the manufacturer of a drug or device. In one case, in 1997, the American Medical Association was criticized for attempting to increase its revenues by signing an endorsement deal with Sunbeam Corporation. The agreement provided that the AMA would be paid for placing its logo on Sunbeam home health care products. Although the AMA stated that the arrangement would benefit patients by encouraging them to monitor their health, the organization was criticized for the conflicts of interest inherent in the deal (SoRelle 1998). Mixed motivations can also be at play when hospitals and medical centers adopt innovations seen as both enhancing medical care and improving the ability to attract patients. Reputation and revenues can improve immensely when a medical institution becomes knows as "the" place for the most up-to-date cancer treatment, for instance. Persuasion from the medical staff can also induce a hospital to provide infrastructure and support for new technologies, such as advanced laser devices, that permit the medical staff to offer advanced procedures. When the large academic hospitals adopt a new treatment modality, competing hospitals are motivated to do the same, out of a desire to meet community needs or, often, because it will help the hospital retain medical staff and preserve their patient base.

A major influence on whether an innovation becomes adopted is the cost of the treatment and the coverage decisions made by public and private insurers. Various health policy studies, along with the experience of pharmaceutical companies, have shown that new medical technologies and expensive drugs disseminate rapidly once they are covered by third-party payers. The only patients with access to new treatments for which no reimbursement is available are a limited population of the relatively wealthy. Insurance coverage decisions have increasingly become a battleground in the current cost-constrained medical environment.

A typical and important case study demonstrating the influence of insurance coverage entails the use of high-dose chemotherapy (HDC, which provides a higher cancer cell kill rate than regular chemotherapy) followed by autologous bone marrow transplant (BMT, which restores the bone marrow tissue destroyed by the high doses of cancer drugs) for women with advanced breast cancer. In the 1980s and 1990s, this treatment was reserved for women who had failed to re- cover on standard cancer treatments and whose prognosis was grim. Based on data from some uncontrolled studies, HDC followed by BMT gained a reputation as the last-ditch survival chance for patients with late-stage breast cancer. Al- though potentially a lifesaver, the treatment was toxic and expensive, costing as much as $200,000. Many insurance companies refused to cover the procedures, claiming that not enough evidence existed to establish efficacy. Despite this lack of coverage, up to 5,000 U.S. women per year in the 1990s received the treatment and it was widely endorsed by cancer center oncologists, who often personally lob- bied insurers to cover treatment costs for their patients. Insurance companies continued to balk and persisted in demands for convincing proof of efficacy.

Finally in 1991, the National Cancer Institute (NCI) sponsored several large randomized controlled trials. Recruitment for these trials went slowly; some on- cologists, considering the treatment effective, declined to ask women to become research subjects if they could afford the treatment. Some prospective enrollees declined out of worry that they risked assignment to the control group receiving conventional treatment. While the research trials were under way, moreover, steady improvements in cancer treatment—both conventional and with BMT— were occurring, making assessment of the BMT treatment a moving target. In addition to any data interpretation difficulties, it would take years for the NCI trials to be completed. In the meantime, insurance companies were being sued for denial of coverage: the best-known lawsuit was brought when Nelene Fox died in 1993 after she had been denied coverage for HDC with BMT by Health Net of California. The jury refused to believe the defendant HMO's claim that treatment coverage was denied because the treatment was experimental. The patient's family was awarded $89.1 million, more than the net worth of the company.[5] The lawyer who obtained this judgment, Mark Hiepler, was the brother of the dead patient, and the experience turned him into a crusader. The traditional view of plaintiff's lawyers is that they discourage medical innovation by filing product liability or malpractice lawsuits. *Fox v. Health Net* is an example of the opposite effect. After this first win, Hiepler's legal advocacy and litigating skills on behalf of other patients who had been denied coverage prompted several third-party payers to begin covering this breast cancer treatment.

Meanwhile, however, commentary in the medical literature began to question the efficacy of the treatment for late-stage disease, and some practitioners were starting to withhold HDC with BMT. Doubts were eased when one small, 90-patient, study from South Africa showed that HDC followed by BMT was more effective than a conventional breast cancer treatment regimen. The study was judged sufficiently credible by oncologists performing BMT, leading to claims that the treatment should be adopted as standard and covered by insurance companies. Some insurance companies continued to resist, however, and more lawsuits were lost. But then, in 1999, four larger trials failed to show that HDC followed by BMT was better than conventional treatment for breast cancer (Staudmauer et al. 2000). The new data caused many oncologists to stop offering the treatment, and demand for the procedure dropped. So, naturally, did the number of lawsuits claiming wrongful denial of coverage, and denial increased. Decisions to deny coverage gained further credence after the discovery that the South African investigators had falsified their study data (Weiss 2001). Since then, HDC followed by BMT has been offered under experimental protocols. This narrative illustrates how difficult it is to establish the efficacy of new treatments, and it also shows what a powerful influence insurance coverage can have on the dissemination of medical technology.

Another factor that can broaden public acceptance of medical innovations is demand by patients and their advocacy groups. Advocacy organizations have become a potent force in influencing physicians to provide treatments, insurance companies to cover those treatments, and legislators to pass laws supporting access to them. In fact, physicians, insurers, and legislators were all targeted by breast cancer activists in the 1990s on behalf of HDC with BMT. One example of their success occurred just after publication of the first South African study, when the Minnesota legislature required health plans doing business in the state to pay for HDC with autologous BMT (Minnesota Statutes 62A.309).

In generating public acceptance of medical innovations, it is difficult to underestimate the impact of access to the Internet as a force in the dissemination of information. Websites abound at which patients can learn about all manner of treatments, both standard and experimental. They can also learn on line how to pressure medical plans to cover treatments and which legislators to lobby—all of which enhances the ability of individuals to advocate for access to new treatments.

Eventually, because of some or all of these processes and influences, innovative treatments can reach a high level of professional and public acceptance without having been evaluated in rigorously controlled clinical trials. Choosing to innovate in this way is sometimes influenced by the reasons for avoiding the research route. Among these reasons are: the concern that a study of the innovation would not be approved by the research IRB;[6] unwillingness to comply with the burdens of the IRB approval and oversight processes; lack of funds and other resources; the suspicion that research will reveal flaws in the application of the technology; and the desire to keep the innovation private to prevent others from usurping the idea. It is also argued (with some justification) that hospital peer review committees and physician credentialing processes give innovative practices enough scrutiny to ensure that adequate patient protections are in place and that unreasonable risks are not taken when innovative treatments are used. That assurance may break down, however, when no one challenges a powerful physician intent on proceeding with a treatment others find worrisome.

A strong case in favor of forgoing the research route is when an innovation is obviously the best option available to treat a particular condition. It is easy to see that Dr. Upton, in the preceding example, would be reluctant to subject his future use of leeches to a randomized controlled trial in which the provision of his treatment or an alternative would be determined by the randomization schedule of the study protocol. Given the success of the treatment, however, he might well decide that withholding leeching in a similar situation would be unethical. Another argument for bypassing the research route is that clinical observation and experience often provide a faster and less costly route to providing patients with needed medical treatments. The history of the development of propranolol is an example of how an informal and unregulated process of innovation in the practice of medicine has served patients well. This adrenergic beta blocker was originally approved by the FDA for use in arrhythmias and angina. Gradually, physicians who were careful observers of the how the drug behaved tried using it for other conditions, such as hypertension and migraine, with good results. Propranolol is now used beneficially in more than twenty medical conditions, and many of these applications were introduced by physicians willing to engage in an intelligent expansion of use based on observation of the drug's effects. If all of these uses had required formal research (with or without the usual FDA regulatory processes), propranolol would likely remain a drug with limited utility.

On the other hand, in some cases, clinical experience, observational studies, practitioner endorsement, well-intentioned adoption by professional organizations, and public demand are no substitute for careful scientific scrutiny. The use of HDC with BMT in breast cancer is one example. Until the negative studies were reported, thousands of women were treated, many ineffectively and some harmfully, at enormous cost in medical and litigation expense. In some cases, physicians may have suspected that the therapy was not beneficial, but clinical experience alone was insufficient to make that determination. The state of ignorance was prolonged because physicians do not often publish reports of unsuccessful treatments. The kind of medical, insurance, and legal controversies that existed with HDC with BMT for breast cancer demonstrate why randomized controlled trials may be necessary to show that a treatment is not entitled to the confidence physicians have placed in it.

This brings us to the next (but not the last) phase in the life cycle of medical technology: denunciation and death. The discovery that a treatment is not safe or is not effective or that there are safer, more effective, or as good but cheaper alternatives are all common reasons for discarding an established treatment. Such revelations can come about from observation or research. If a gold standard research study shows lack of efficacy or excessive risk, physicians tend to question and then abandon the treatment. Examples where research led to the demise of standard practice interventions include: internal mammary artery ligation for angina, routine tonsillectomy, prophylactic use of portal-caval shunts for cirrhosis patients at risk for esophageal bleeding, radical mastectomy in breast cancer, bloodletting (although not in all countries), lung transplants in children with cystic fibrosis, routine circumcision, arthroscopic surgery for osteoarthritis of the knee, reliance on antacids to treat stomach ulcers, the use of clofibrate to lower cholesterol, exchange transfusions for newborns with high serum bilirubin, and routine use of electronic fetal monitors.

But, even solid research debunking of a medical treatment does not always result in its demise. Physicians can be so committed to treatments that adverse research findings will not sway them. Doctors whose medical practice depends on income from the treatment in question are likewise reluctant to abandon it. Both groups can find methodological flaws to cast doubt on the findings of new studies, and these objections may be credible, because perfect studies are difficult to design. In other cases, studies, even good ones, can be discounted because they were conducted by physicians with a vested interest in their outcome. The nature of the treatment is also relevant: it is easier to abandon the prescribing of a drug than, for instance, a surgical procedure that requires the use of specialized machines into which the hospital invested significant money. Reluctance to jettison a treatment is also higher when there are no alternatives available.

For all of these reasons and more, it can take several controlled trials showing lack of efficacy or safety to overcome years of positive practical experience supported by convincing anecdotal reports. Also, what purports to be the definitive study of the effects of a treatment may be undercut by other studies that produced conflicting results. In the years of uncertainty while new studies are being designed, conducted, published, and analyzed, physicians' clinical experience determines whether a treatment or procedure remains part of the medical arsenal. Patients can be another factor in prolonging a treatment's longevity when they plead to continue a discredited treatment. This argument is often respected, because data from aggregate studies are an imperfect predictor of how well a treatment will work in an individual patient.

An instructive case study of the influence of patient demand is the randomized controlled trial involving menopausal hormone replacement therapy (HRT). Menopausal HRT (usually combinations of estrogen and progestins) had been prescribed for decades in the belief that it relieved the symptoms of menopause (hot flashes, mood swings, insomnia, stiffness, vaginal dryness, weight changes, etc.) and offered long-term prevention of cardiovascular illness, osteoporosis, mental deterioration, and other age-related changes. These beliefs, based primarily on observational reports and uncontrolled studies, resulted in widespread prescribing of HRT among the two million women who experience menopause each year. This popularity persisted despite the understanding that risks, including increased cancer risk, were associated with the practice. Then, in 2002, a large randomized placebo-controlled trial called the Women's Health Initiative (WHI) (Writing Group for the Women's Health Initiative Investigators 2002) was reported. This study had been designed to determine conclusively whether HRT was beneficial for postmenopausal women. The data showed that, although menopausal symptoms may have been controlled, the therapy was more likely to lead to increased risk of breast cancer, heart attack, stroke, and pulmonary embolism while failing to offer some of the benefits previously attributed to the regimen. At first, the study report caused widespread abandonment of the use of HRT. It appeared that the long-term use of postmenopausal HRT was dead.

Then, after years of reassessment, arguments emerged that provided a different perspective on the interpretation of the data. In particular, it was pointed out that the study conclusions did not apply to women outside of the age range of the subjects, women who had started HRT earlier in life, or women who took different doses of HRT than those given in the study or for different amounts of time. Also, it took a while for the magnitude of the HRT risk to sink in—for women to realize that the absolute risk of harm was very small (e.g., 38 cases of breast cancer per year for every 10,000 women who received HRT and 30 for those on placebo). These reassessments generated arguments against the widespread abandonment of HRT, which were augmented by the pleas of patients who, having stopped taking HRT on their doctor's recommendation, had experienced significant misery with the return of menopausal symptoms. As a result, doctors were persuaded to restart treatment for many women (Ockene et al. 2005). Pharmaceutical companies, which had watched the sales of their HRT drugs plummet, contributed to the reassessment of the WHI trial data and obliged the medical community and patients by providing lower-dose drugs for those who wanted to reduce their risk of side effects while continuing treatment. More studies (as this book was going to press, new studies were being reported) will likely help us understand how these drugs fit into the overall management of postmenopausal health. The treatment may even be fully reestablished, albeit in modified form. It is also likely that the WHI study will prompt attempts to discover new forms of hormonal treatment that reduce the identified risks.

If HRT returns, in some form, to anything like its earlier popularity, it will provide an illustration of the last phase of medical innovation, one that brings us full cycle. That phase is resurrection. Often, a committed group of practitioners come to believe that a particular therapy failed for lack of a modification, for instance, or because of inappropriate selection of patients. These physicians will continue to modify the therapy through practical use or through research, either of which can reestablish the treatment as accepted medical care. This kind of rejuvenation is likeliest when the therapy addresses an important unmet medical need, when physicians believe they know the reason for treatment failure, and/or when the medical theory behind the therapy is highly credible. Innovation can feed innovation: new developments can resurrect a stagnant medical intervention, as when immunosuppressive drugs allowed organ transplantation surgery to flourish. Sometimes the need to control health care costs can also prompt a reassessment of discarded treatments. Because most new therapies are more expensive than the ones they hope to replace, reassessment of older, cheaper treatments may be undertaken to determine if the higher costs of new therapies are justified.

Cost issues explain why randomized controlled trials and meta-analyses were conducted in the late 1990s comparing older, low-cost thiazide diuretics with newer antihypertension drugs that cost sometimes more than ten times as much. These studies reestablished a place of primary importance for diuretics in the treatment of hypertension (Wright, Lee, and Chambers 1999). A similar resurrection is now being attempted for HDC with BMT for breast cancer. Practitioners have continued to modify the procedure by abandoning the use of bone marrow and substituting a procedure in which stem cells harvested from bone marrow are reinfused after high-dose cancer drug therapy. The new procedure, called autologous stem cell transplant, is now being offered to breast cancer patients under research protocols (Farquhar et al. 2005).

Another interesting medical treatment resurrection occurred with prefrontal lobotomy,[7] the surgical procedure used on patients with disabling psychiatric conditions before the discovery of effective medicinal treatments. This procedure was used on tens of thousands of patients in the United States from the 1930s to the mid-1960s (Valenstein 1986) but was abandoned when it was revealed to be associated with high rates of complication, including intellectual impairment, emotional and personality change, seizure, paralysis, and death. The procedure became publicly unpopular when portrayed as a method of behavior control in the movie *One Flew over the Cuckoo's Nest* and when it was reported that President John F. Kennedy's sister had become permanently incapacitated after the procedure. But, aided by advances in imaging and other medical technologies, proponents of the procedure continued attempts at refinement, believing that more targeted destruction of brain cells offered promise for those patients with severe, refractory depression and obsessive compulsive disorder. As a result, the practice of psychosurgery was reborn with procedures such as cingulotomy, which attempts to ablate very small and specific areas of brain tissue believed to be responsible for the abnormal psychiatric symptoms (Cosgrove and Rauch 2003).[8] Many insurance companies (Aetna 2005) are withholding judgment about coverage for psychosurgical procedures, objecting on several grounds that the studies so far are not persuasive: the study designs are retrospective; the diagnostic systems used vary from study to study; independent clinical raters of safety and efficacy are not always used; the psychosurgical techniques vary; and studies often lack true control groups. Nonetheless, several practitioners at large university medical centers have seen cingulotomy produce the only relief from severe treatment-resistant psychiatric suffering, and they continue to perform and re-

fine their procedures for such patients. An interesting consequence of this innovation resulted when cingulotomy was performed on cancer patients with severe
depression. Because the procedure also resulted in relief of cancer pain, cingulotomy has become accepted as a last-resort treatment for cancer patients with
intractable pain.

Resurrections of innovations have often been examples of the common situation in which medical innovation occurs in several ways at once—some new,
some old, many creating uncertainty about the wisdom of adopting a particular
treatment. While some physicians are conducting research on a new treatment,
others are already offering the treatment in their practice, perhaps refining it as
they use it. Medical innovations often run in parallel; multiple therapies for the
same condition undergo innovation simultaneously, all of them available to patients. This situation leaves treating physicians and patients with the difficult
choice of which to select. Anyone who chooses to research the effectiveness of
new treatments is also left with a choice: whether to compare the treatment to
placebo (i.e., is it better than nothing) or to other treatments.[9] Just as observational studies are not scientific evidence of effectiveness, studies showing that a
treatment is better than placebo say nothing about whether it is better than another therapy. All of these factors complicate the understanding about whether
any particular treatment innovation is medically worthwhile.

A good example of this dilemma is the choice whether to treat coronary artery
disease with medical management, with a surgical procedure, or with various
types of nonsurgical percutaneous intervention to open the affected vessels.[10] All
three have been offered to patients with and without research data to support
their use. Although these three treatment approaches did not arise simultaneously, eventually all three came to exist simultaneously as options. That created a
situation in which patients could receive remarkably different advice depending
on whether they sought treatment from an internist, a cardiac surgeon, or a ra-
diologist skilled at using imaging devices to perform procedures on the body. To
say that there was a difference of opinion about the best way to treat this disease
is an understatement. News of an advance on any front has often renewed turf
battles among the subspecialists about which treatment best served patients.

Once upon a time, there were no turf wars over coronary artery disease. Tra-
ditionally, it was treated solely with medications and (from prevention-oriented
cardiologists) advice to adopt a heart-healthy lifestyle. At first, the only medication available was nitroglycerin, invented in 1847 for use as an explosive. When
early workers handling the substance frequently developed severe headaches,
medical investigations revealed that the headaches were caused by nitroglycerin-

induced vasodilation—a discovery that eventually led to nitroglycerin's use as a coronary vasodilator for patients with angina from blocked coronary blood vessels.[11] Although nitroglycerin was useful, its limitations stimulated the development of other drugs, often used in combination with nitroglycerin and each other. These others are now many and include cholesterol-lowering medications, antiplatelet agents (to reduce the risk of blood clots), glycoprotein IIb–IIIa inhibitors and antithrombin drugs (to reduce the risk of blood clots), beta-blockers (to decrease heart rate and lower oxygen use by the heart), calcium-channel blockers (to relax the coronary and systemic arteries to reduce the workload for the heart), and new antihypertension drugs such as ACE inhibitors. The use of these drugs was generally supported by clinical studies and FDA approval. With such an arsenal of drugs, coronary artery disease can often be well-controlled if the patient is compliant and the monitoring for efficacy and side effects is diligent.

While advances were being made on the medication front, surgeons were experimenting with techniques to open blocked coronary arteries.[12] This work proceeded as surgical innovation, without much oversight or regulation, and literature reports were largely observational. One review counted seventy-five papers in the medical literature in 1970, all of which reported positive results of coronary artery surgery and were based on uncontrolled observation. In that same year, there were exactly two controlled studies, both showing that the surgeries were ineffective. In the meantime, one type of coronary artery surgery, coronary artery bypass grafting (CABG),[13] became a favored procedure for treating coronary artery disease, and this development led to less reliance on medical management. Additional encouragement came from the surgeons themselves, who had a powerful interest in promoting the use of surgical approaches to this common disease. Then in 1972, the Veterans Administration Cooperative Group began an eighteen-year study comparing CABG with medical management of coronary artery disease in more than six hundred patients, with measures that included survival, angina symptoms, exercise tolerance, and postinfarction mortality. Preliminary data from this study were first published in 1975 and showed that the surgery group fared better. Then, eleven-year data came out in the early 1980s showing that the initial surgical benefits had started to fade and that survival, angina relief, and exercise tolerance over a longer term were comparable to those achieved with medical treatment. After eighteen years of follow-up, the final results showed that bypass surgery was effective in reducing early mortality only in patients with a poor natural disease history. Otherwise, the benefits of CABG surgery on survival, angina symptoms, and postinfarction mortality were transient, lasting fewer than eleven years. The benefits began to diminish after five years, when graft closure accelerated. An exception was that there was no survival ben-efit at any time for low-risk patients who had had a good initial prognosis with medical therapy. Regardless of the patient's risk category, surgery also did not re-duce the incidence of myocardial infarction or the combined incidence of infarc-ton or death. (Veterans Affairs Coronary Artery Bypass Surgery Cooperative Study Group 1992).

Throughout the years when these results were being reported, the use of CABG procedures continued to increase. In the early 1980s, when the VA Coop-erative Group data started showing a lack of benefit from surgery, CABG surger-ies were performed on more than 100,000 patients per year, with most of the $2 billion annual costs being covered by public and private medical insurers. By this time, observational reports on the procedure (showing mostly positive out-comes) outnumbered the reports from randomized controlled trials by about 100:1 a difference attributed to the cost and difficulty of designing and conducting randomized controlled trials on cardiac surgical procedures and of persuading patients to join a study in which they might be randomly assigned to the non-surgery group. This situation led many surgeons to conclude that it was appro-priate to offer CABG procedures outside of research protocols, based on the pre-ponderance of the observational reports and the belief that it was unethical to withhold the innovation from patients until the completion of randomized con-trolled trials. Nevertheless, the final data from the VA Cooperative Group did not settle the matter. As with many long-term studies, by the time the randomized controlled trial was completed and reported, the conclusions were difficult to incorporate into medical and surgical practice. Both the bypass procedure and medical management had changed over the intervening years, and belief in the effectiveness and perfectibility of CABG surgery prevailed despite the Veterans Administration study results demonstrating that the procedure offered no long-term benefits over medication. A small, skeptical minority of physicians continue to ask for more randomized controlled trials, but the procedure has undergone what historians of technology call "path dependence"—once established, a tech-nology and those who do it well become settled in and difficult to dislodge.

Lagging behind the medical and surgical approaches to coronary artery dis-ease and in response to their limitations, various percutaneous coronary inter-ventions were being developed, the most popular of which was percutaneous transluminal coronary angioplasty (PTCA, also called balloon angioplasty).[14] The first PTCA was performed around 1977. After that, the procedure quickly under-went modification, greatly improving outcomes and reducing the need for riskier and more expensive open heart surgeries such as CABG. And, as with CABG, observational reports of success and modifications that improved results encouraged surgeons to adopt the procedure. Currently, surgeons can complete an angioplasty procedure in ninety minutes compared to the two to four hours required for open bypass surgery. Patients can be discharged in one day instead of five or six days, and recovery takes only one week compared to four to six weeks for open surgery. The improvements also resulted in major cost savings, with an angioplasty currently costing less than half the $50,000 usually charged for open-heart surgery. Moreover, there is general agreement that PTCA, once mastered by the surgeon, can significantly improve the quality of life for many patients who require surgery for the condition. An additional factor spurring dissemination of PTCA is that reimbursement for the procedure has been relatively easy to obtain. These successes and influences have made coronary angioplasty the most common medical intervention in the world. One million of the procedures were performed in 1997, and the number increased to about two million by 2001, according to the PTCA Anniversary Project (www.ptca.org).

The increasing reliance on coronary angioplasty, however, has not been trouble free. Experience with the procedure revealed an unexpectedly high requirement for second procedures when restenosis occurred (the blood vessels closing off again). These reoperations increase both the risk and the total costs of angioplasty. Continued innovation was applied to this problem, and most surgeons now insert intracoronary stents after angioplasty, to keep the blood vessels open, preventing restenosis and the need for a second operation. The first models of these stents also failed in a significant number of patients, but new stents were introduced that were impregnated with drugs intended to prevent the blood clots that contributed to restenosis. As this book went to press, news about problems with these drug-eluting stents was surfacing, no doubt prompting surgeons to devise ways to further refine both the procedure and the surgical devices.

Once all three of these approaches to the treatment of coronary artery disease had developed to the point of viability, the question became which to use in a patient. It was clear that each had shortcomings and that there were significant cost differences among them. Because of the huge numbers of doctors and patients who need to choose among these three options, studies were begun of their relative utility (Brorsson, Bernstein, and Herlitz 1999). These studies will undoubtedly be plagued with the same problems seen with the VA Cooperative Group study—namely, that controlled clinical trials based on long-term outcomes are difficult to initiate and the results are often difficult to interpret. In the meantime, more surgical and medical practice innovations will undoubtedly occur in an effort to improve all three. The chapter of this book dealing with surgical innovations introduces a new addition on this innovative path.

The processes of development and refining of medical and surgical innovations described above supply insights into what to expect with innovations now arriving on the scene. These include: the microminiaturization of surgical tools, expanded use of laser and radio-frequency tissue-cutting devices, fetal surgery, diagnostic machine improvements, disease gene testing, bioengineered animal and human tissues, gene therapies, advanced protein-based medicines, drugs from bioengineered plants, stem cell therapies, nanotechnology-based medicines, and advanced medical information technologies.[15] Experiences with these technologies are likely to mirror the phases of development and dissemination traveled by other technologies. Our hope as we discuss those journeys is that the history of earlier and existing technologies, together with the case studies we present, will add to the understanding of how medical innovation comes about and is deployed and of the broader consequences of choosing one path or another along the innovation process.

These broader consequences are a primary focus of our book. In its formative stages, innovation necessarily takes the medical scientist and clinician into poorly charted territories, where unknown and unintended consequences are a chronic reality. Medical progress is never risk free, and real harms are among the consequences of medical innovation—harms to people (both sick and healthy), to the medical profession, to payers and insurers, and even to society. Sometimes these harms are apparent immediately, as when some of the first coronary angioplasty patients died soon after the procedure; some risks materialize slightly later, as when restenosis was discovered months after angioplasty procedures; and other harms have taken much longer to become manifest, as in the cases of Guillain-Barré syndrome following the 1976 swine flu immunization program and when the daughters of women who had taken DES developed gynecologic cancers. Other failures also harm the physician, as when the integrity of a physician, evidently innovating within a research protocol, was called into question because a relatively healthy teenager with a rare genetic disorder died during a pioneering gene therapy experiment.[16]

Harmful outcomes, especially if any lack of diligence in patient protection is involved, can undermine the public's willingness to trust medical technology, or even the medical profession itself. Public trust is weakened when doctors are perceived as using patients as guinea pigs (as they were with the first animal-to-human heart transplants); when patients' consent is poorly informed (e.g., the inadequate disclosure and consent procedures used in early in vitro fertilization procedures); when costly treatments are shown to lack benefit (e.g., bone marrow transplants in late-stage breast cancer); when medical privacy is breached (e.g., early tissue banks were linked to patients' medical records without consent); and when unanticipated social harms result (e.g., some early genetic testing that revealed a predisposition to disease ruined patients' sense of well-being and disqualified them from insurance coverage or employment).

Trust can also be eroded by the high costs of medical innovations in their early stages, revealing that access to cutting-edge medicine is available mostly to the wealthy or fully insured and that some innovations in medicine will unsustainably increase the cost of health care. For example, hospitals started to limit the use of drug-eluting stents to high-risk patients when stent popularity combined with low reimbursement rates threatened hospital budgets.

Finally, public confidence may be compromised by perceived violation of a variety of ethical, moral, or religious standards that people may apply to different forms of medical innovation. Among these subjects of concern are technologies used to extend life beyond an assumed "natural" course, those making possible novel methods of baby-making, the harvesting of stem cells from human embryos for therapeutic purposes, and pharmaceutical interventions that may change personality or enhance physical capacity or cognitive skills. The last have been of particular concern because they raise the issue of use not for treatment but for enhancement purposes. The prospects for new technological interventions and novel pharmaceuticals and other medical innovations are now widely publicized, and these early reports often shape the public's attitudes toward the technology. The response commonly involves uncertainty, for today's rapid pace of technological advance allows people little time to understand the implications of new developments. Public perception of medical innovation is thus often understandably conflicted. While new technology is highly valued, it carries with it a certain level of moral and social anxiety.

This anxiety may also be part of the generalized uncertainty in times of rapid change. It is very difficult to predict the consequences of novelty; moreover, the consequences of new technology now have a far broader reach than they did in the past. We understand that medical innovation brings with it prospective benefits, but many of us need to ask what level of individual sacrifice is justifiable to establish the new thing in the domain of standard of care. Public ambivalence about the commercialization of new drugs, devices, or procedures complicates the picture by raising questions about cost, access, and distributive justice. These sources of uncertainty provide a background for a number of pressing questions that are more specific: Are new medical technologies being deployed responsibly? Are patients being exploited during their development? Do serious conflicts of interest exist that impair the physician's judgment? Are the professionalism of medicine and the well-being of patients being served in the best possible ways? For those who think about these questions, there is value in the careful examination of the issues addressed in this book: the consequences of innovation for stakeholders, the nature of benefit and risk, professional duty, patients' rights, conflicts of interest, and social and distributive justice. The prospects for our collective future health surely seem brighter because of new medical technologies that can prevent disease, prolong life, and enhance the benefit and reduce the risk from medical treatment. But public concerns about how we got here and where our new abilities will take us continue to be a part of the ongoing, often agonizing debate about the future of the health care system in the United States. The innovative process is built into medical science; it has its own set of economic and prestige incentives, and they are not going to go away. Our purpose here has been to examine some questions about how innovation develops and how it is deployed. Thinking through these questions, we believe, is an important part of deciding what kind of health care system we want.

CHAPTER ONE

Distinguishing Innovative Medical Practice from Research

Before we address any of the ethical issues associated with innovation in medical technology and whether it should proceed as practice or as research, we must ask a fundamental definitional question: What is innovative medical practice and what is research? The problem of distinguishing the two was thoroughly considered in the United States more than thirty years ago. In 1974, Congress, reacting to reports of unethical treatment and abuse of human subjects,[1] passed the National Research Act and created the National Commission for the Protection of Human Subjects of Biomedical and Behavioral Research. The commission was charged with identifying the basic ethical principles that should underlie the conduct of biomedical and behavioral research on humans and with developing guidelines to assure that such research is conducted in accordance with those principles. In carrying out this charge, the commission was to identify the boundary between biomedical and behavioral research and the accepted and routine practice of medicine. Several preliminary and background papers were submitted to assist the commission with this boundary establishment; those papers are cited in the notes to this chapter.

Robert J. Levine, chief of clinical pharmacology at Yale University, who was asked to staff the commission, wrote the preliminary paper on the boundaries between research and accepted and routine practice (Levine 1979). This paper was sent out to several experts (internists, surgeons, psychiatrists, philosophers, and lawyers among them) for critical comment and was then submitted to the commissioners to assist their deliberations. From the beginning, it was clear that Levine and some of the commentators found it difficult to identify clear boundaries between research and practice. A great deal of health care professional activity had elements of both, Levine had recorded. What's more, benefits seemed to result from combining the two. However, in order to develop protections for the subjects of research, the commission was required to make a distinction between research and medical practice, because the regulations they were to write were to apply only to research.

Levine first tackled the distinction between a patient and a research subject. A patient, he wrote, is the client of the physician and should be able to safely assume that the physician is acting solely in the client's best interests. The resulting duty of care means that, even though ultimate decision making rests with the patient, he or she should feel safe in delegating some decisions to the physician. A research subject, in contrast, is a person experimented on and observed by the physician. The research physician has an interest in the subject's welfare but may have an even a greater interest in collecting data to serve a larger set of patient interests. As a consequence, subjects should feel less secure in entrusting decision making to the research physician. Based on this understanding, Levine then explored ways to identify boundaries between research and practice when the doctor's role had elements of both.

One way to make distinctions was to analyze physician intent. When the clear intent was to apply the best available therapies to yield the most medical good for the patient, Levine called this the "pure practice of medicine." If the physician intended to develop new knowledge not *primarily* for the benefit of the patient, that could be defined as research. Usually, but not necessarily, a research intent is evidenced by a written protocol. In cases where there is no written protocol, matters proceed less formally. There may be a serendipitous discovery, a finding in one patient that the physician then attempts to apply to similar patients, for example, when a drug benefits a patient unexpectedly and the physician then prescribes it for others with the same condition, or when a physician develops a lab test to measure a substance thought to be associated with a disease and then uses it as a marker in all of his patients suspected of having the disease. The natural history of a disease is sometimes discovered in this way, as with the discovery of the biomarker for malignant carcinoid. Retrospectively, it seems as if the investigator intended to look for this marker, whereas it was really an exploration rather like Darwin's; as a result, this kind of experiment is sometimes called a "Voyage of the Beagle."

Levine next suggested that the boundary issue could also be addressed through a social system approach, considering the views and judgments of groups such as peer reviewers, IRBs, and regulatory agencies, all of which customarily make distinctions between research and accepted medical practice. They may have the authority to disapprove certain treatments, but individual physicians do not always agree with the group's conclusions and may persevere in using the treatment.

Another possible boundary marker involves the complexity of the physician-patient interaction. In cases where several treatments are provided, some may be therapy and some may be more like research. A physician who is treating a patient for an unusual disease manifestation may conduct extra lab tests in the hope of identifying something useful—and possibly worth publishing. Levine suggested that physicians in such cases inform the patient which of the activities constitute research. That would enable the patient to know that the lab tests are not primarily intended to improve his or her health and free the patient to reject the tests without prejudicing his or her access to health care or incurring extra bills. If the interaction with the physician is simpler, as when one drug is being used to treat a disease, a major boundary question involves whether the treatment is accepted or the best available. Approval by the FDA can sometimes set the boundary between research and treatment and also determine whether the treatment is deemed "accepted." But the FDA's determination may not survive strong differences of opinion in the medical community as to which treatments are "accepted" and "best available" or the "drug of choice." This exposes two boundary problems. The first is the boundary between what is research and what is practice (if a drug is not accepted, its use can seem like research). The second, determined by practice, is what is considered accepted or "best available" and what isn't. The problem becomes more complex when there is no standard-setting body—such as there is for drugs. For instance, Levine noted that there is no FDA equivalent for surgery, invasive diagnostic techniques (e.g., biopsies, catheterizations), diagnostic and therapeutic devices (some are only lightly regulated), radioisotopes, radiation and other physical forms of therapy, and behavioral approaches as in psychotherapy.[2] Levine proposes that some mechanism be established allowing these treatments to be classified as rejected, approved, accepted, safe, or efficacious.

Levine then turned to a discussion of innovative therapy, the concept for which was established by Dr. Francis Moore (see Introduction) in his article, "Therapeutic Innovation: Ethical Boundaries in the Initial Clinical Trials of New Drugs and Surgical Procedures" (1969). In addition to being a new modality, an innovation can be an old modality used in a new way, in a new dose, or in combination with other new or old modalities. What innovative treatments have in common is that they have not been sufficiently tested to meet peer or regulatory standards for acceptance or approval. They can be simple treatments or can be used with mixed therapeutic and research intent. Levine asserted that, ideally, innovative therapies should be presented as research—as experimental—although he did not recommend that new regulatory bodies be established to govern the process of medical innovation. He did, however, suggest that the FDA model could be helpful in defining innovative treatments (akin to drugs in Phase II or III research), in determining how research should proceed (animals first, then increasing numbers of patients), and in deciding when it is appropriate to abandon an innovative treatment (as judged through surveillance that could recommend full or limited withdrawal or a requirement for warning). Levine expressed a preference for testing new treatments only during the process of innovation, not after use had become established, to avoid the difficulties associated with conducting research on firmly established even though possibly harmful treatments. His view was based on the experience the FDA had in reviewing after the fact drugs introduced to the market between 1938 and 1962, hoping to establish if they were effective for their designated indications. Although that study, called DESI (Drug Efficacy Study Implementation), was supposedly finished by 1969 (National Academy of Sciences 1969), efficacy data were still missing for many of those "grandfathered in" drugs. In the late 1970s, the agency was still being ordered by judges to finish the study. This situation is hardly surprising: once therapies are considered accepted and routine, few physicians and patients are willing to engage in research to determine the efficacy and safety that they assume exists. Finally, Levine recommended that exceptions to requiring systematic study of innovative treatments include situations in which patients with life-threatening illnesses require emergency treatment and no other reasonable treatment options exist. However, in such cases, physicians who use innovative treatments as medical practice should understand that they can be held accountable retrospectively to the hospital board or the institutional review board.

The responses of the expert commentators to Levine's paper were mixed. With regard to using physician intent to delineate research from medical practice, some commentators were uneasy about leaving physicians to self-report on what they originally intended when they innovated. As one advisor wrote to the commission, "Intent is a rather slender reed upon which to build public policy . . . ever since Freud, at least, we have learned to question even self-assessment of intent, no matter how sincerely or tenaciously held" (Goldiamond 1979, p. 14-4). Not only is there no objective measure of intent, but also motives may be hidden if the physician seeks to avoid the time and cost burdens of research and instead treat the patient quickly. Self-interest could also influence the physician's retrospective statements about intent if he were accused of conducting research without IRB approval or proper consent.

The subject of intent was most prominently addressed in the paper to the commission authored by the commenting lawyer, John Robertson (Robertson 1979), now a professor at the University of Texas at Austin School of Law. Robertson identified two problems with using physician intent to distinguish between research and practice. The first

concerns a distinction between general and specific intent. In law one is often held to intend the natural and probable consequence of one's act, even though one specifically intended or aimed only to do the act producing those consequences [cite omitted]. Since a particular therapeutic use of an innovative therapy may naturally yield knowledge concerning use with other patients, one might argue that a general intent to use the therapy should be treated as an intent to derive knowledge for other uses, merely because such knowledge is a likely or natural and probable consequence of its use. Usually a physician will know that such knowledge will result, so that the possibility of a nonpatient benefit might, albeit subconsciously, influence his decision to use the therapy, even though at the time of use he specifically intends only therapy and benefit to the patient. However, if an interest conflicting with the patient's operates only on the subconscious level, it does not differ from the physician's interests in extra income, time, etc. that may conflict with patient interests in situations of ordinary therapy and which arguably deserve no special protection. The strongest case for treating the general intent to use an innovative therapy as equivalent to a specific intent to acquire knowledge beyond the patient's best interests would exist in the first use of a drug or new surgical procedure. Here the development of knowledge is inevitable, and here it is likely that the intent to gain new knowledge is strong, or at least equivalent to the therapeutic intent. (Robertson 1979, pp. 16-36–16-37)

Robertson went on to say that a second problem with an intent criterion for differentiation was its implementation. Any system in place to review and approve research would necessarily depend on the good faith of physicians to overtly acknowledge their intent to conduct research on patients and voluntarily submit to review and oversight. Such a system would be subject to abuse, because some physicians would have an incentive to emphasize a therapeutic purpose even though research played the dominant role in their motivation. Also, there could be no sanctions for physicians who failed to submit to a research review process, because intent can never be proved.

Other commentators believed that the intent of the patient/subject was a more important factor. To preserve patient trust and well-being, they said, patients who intend to obtain medical help should not be treated by physicians who have both scientific and therapeutic intentions or whose intentions are unclear because the only treatments available are experimental (London and Klerman 1979). Commentators concerned about the congruence of physician and patient intent felt that if the physician intends to perform research, it *is* research, and human subject protections should apply, such as peer oversight and requirements for full and uncoerced consent.

Conversely, not all that is intended by the physician to be therapy is therapy. On this point, the commentators' distinction was based on whether the therapy was routine and accepted. If so, it was therapy; if not, it was research. These commentators went on to say that the focus should therefore be placed not on intent but on demonstrating that a treatment is safe and effective.

> We can attack the problem of boundaries meaningfully by recognizing that the practical problem is that many therapeutic methods are well intended, but poorly established (in terms of safety, efficacy, and economy). One cannot demonstrate the efficacy of a therapy in terms of the intentions of its proponents, because nice guys, in addition to finishing last, may propose ineffective treatments. And they may even propose harmful therapies with the best of intentions. No more can a therapy be considered routine and acceptable on the basis of authority. Only evidence will do. (London and Klerman 1979, p. 15-5)

The risks involved with untested therapies were significant enough, some commentators believed, not to leave patients' fates in the hands of the well-intentioned physician. Some objective evidence was required. A treatment used by Dr. Benjamin Rush (1745–1813) was cited by one commentator as an example of why physician intent should not be relied on in determining whether a therapy is considered standard or experimental. Dr. Rush was one of the founders of American medicine. Although an eminent physician, politician, philosopher, and social reformer, the zeal and determination with which he advocated a type of therapy involving severe bloodletting and purging eventually ruined his medical career. During the yellow fever epidemics of the 1790s, Dr. Rush was energetic in ministering to the sick, but although no one doubted his good intentions, his treatments were alleged to have caused more deaths among his patients than the disease would have. Criticism against Dr. Rush became so strong that he was forced to leave his medical career (North 2000). Focusing on this cautionary tale tempted some commentators to conclude that the intent problem could be solved only by moving from subjective intent to an objective standard, that is, by requiring that evidence determine what is therapy and what is research. That generated an obvious question: How much evidence is necessary to classify a treatment as within the realm of acceptable medical practice? And that returns us to the initial question: Where can we locate the boundary between research and practice?

If intent was not suitable for distinguishing research from medical practice, what was? Some commentators (Goldiamond 1979; London and Klerman 1979) concluded that, save when the physician is operating under an IRB-approved research protocol, nothing seemed to serve as a clear-cut marker. Among the long list of possibilities suggested by Goldiamond, London, and Klerman were these: what the patient intends; who has asked for help from whom (in treatment, the patient seeks out the doctor, to improve health, and in research the physician seeks out the patient); how far the treatment is from standard practice; how much information is available about the treatment; whether the patient benefited from the intervention; who pays whom for what; the consequences of the interaction; whether the outcome of the intervention is certain; whether a granting agency would fund the activity as research; how a peer review committee would view the activity; and whether the doctor decides to collect and analyze outcomes and publish results. The commentators could envision scenarios in which any one of these markers could indicate that research was taking place or that medical treatment was being provided, or both.

Making the distinction between research and practice was difficult for other reasons. Some physicians advising the commission believed that variability among patients and in the manifestation of diseases and injuries required physicians to deviate frequently from customary practice. What should that kind of medical adaptation be called? One approach would classify any deviation from accepted medical practice as research. Others felt that this approach would unacceptably sweep most medical practice into the realm of research. Not only would medical care be stifled but also patients would be deprived of the skillful adaptive practices that further patient health. As one commentator wrote, "Every surgical procedure is in a sense an experiment . . . and innovations are being made daily as an individual surgeon finds improved results with specific changes in operative technique" (Sabiston 1979, p. 17-7). There was so much crossover, some argued, that clear distinctions between the two entities were impossible when the physician was changing practice to adapt to patient variability. Still others suggested a distinction among three types of physician activity—research, the routine and accepted practice of medicine, and innovative medicine. This last term can be defined as a departure from the routine and accepted practice of medicine, producing outcomes that can be tested by means short of randomized controlled trials.

An additional difficulty in addressing this boundary question is that the commission was examining the boundaries between research and the "accepted and routine practice of medicine." Most commentators recommended a healthy skepticism, to avoid the assumption that "accepted and routine" was the same as safe and effective. One respondent, a psychiatrist, cited examples such as classical psychoanalysis, encounter group therapy, marathon group therapy, aversion conditioning, and psychosurgery—all of which were accepted and routine to many practitioners despite never having been validated as safe and effective and even after having been rejected by other groups of practitioners. The charge to the commission, said that commentator,

> totally ignored the reality that the present "accepted and routine practice of medicine" is frequently less than adequate in many sections of the United States. Thus, "accepted and routine practice" of medicine by some physicians includes techniques that have not been scientifically proved in a valid manner and could, therefore, be considered research. In many cases, the "accepted and routine practice of medicine" deviates from the "intelligent" practice of medicine to such an extent that the ignorant physician is actually conducting research without the realization that he is utilizing unproved techniques in the treatment of his patient. . . . Perhaps more appropriate terminology might have been, "the boundaries between biomedical or behavioral research involving human subjects and the competent practice of medicine based upon scientifically valid experimentation." (Gallant 1979, p. 13-1)

With this suggested terminology, the commentator was setting boundaries that, though clear enough, might have been meant for a world he did not believe existed. His definition left out a large segment of physician activity that was neither research nor treatment based on valid research. The commentator's solution was essentially to upgrade the practice of medicine through a system that would evaluate the safety and effectiveness of all treatments. He suggested "Local Extraordinary Treatment Committees" consisting of impartial legal, statistical, and physician advisors to validate treatments that had been subjected to published placebo-controlled research. If such data did not exist, the treatment could be allowed to continue—but only temporarily and with the fully informed consent of the patient—until it could be researched under IRB approval. Whether the treatment was ultimately accepted or rejected would depend on the published research findings, and appeals of the local committee's decisions could be made to a regional and then a national committee. Such a system, argued the commentator, would best serve patient welfare because only safe and effective treatments would be offered. These committees could also approve the use of untested innovative treatment in situations in which available scientifically valid treatments had failed. (An example given was the use of a dose higher than recommended by the FDA of a medication for a patient with drug-refractory schizophrenia.)

This proposal naturally troubled others, even those who believed that there was inadequate supervision and control over innovative medical practice. Patients need timely access to treatment, and there weren't enough practitioners to staff the medical practice review committees (that kind of shortage is now commonly experienced by IRBs). Others felt that the policy would amount to an intrusion on the practice of medicine and an undue burden on medical innovation. Even if the risks of an innovative therapy were higher than standard therapy and more akin to the risks inherent in research, some felt that there was no need for new controls to reduce or minimize the risks. They suggested that the risk-reducing incentives of tort liability and peer review systems would suffice, either as they existed or with some enhancements. One commentator pointed out that most physicians appreciate the risks inherent in using innovative treatments and that the prospect of liability or professional censure provides sufficient incentive to be careful about obtaining consent and assuring that the patient has a reasonable chance of benefiting. If these incentives are considered too weak, perhaps physicians could be subject to stricter liability or be entitled to fewer legal defenses when patients are injured from innovative therapies. However, implementing either of these legal sanctions would most likely deter physicians from innovating. As an alternative, special risk disclosures might be imposed for innovative treatments, but those might cause patients to decline novel treatments that could help them. Improving physician peer review or medical quality-control systems might also prompt innovating physicians to make better risk-benefit decisions and more complete disclosures to patients. These improvements could include enhanced education, more precise norms and criteria for use of innovative therapies, and more peer monitoring. Although they may improve patient care, these alternatives also pose problems of insufficient efficacy, high cost, and enforcement difficulties (Robertson 1979).

The commission's response to the debate and commentary about the boundaries between research and practice became a part of its report on protections for human subjects, called the Belmont Report. In this report, the commission offered guidance on the definition of *clinical research*—"an activity designed to test an hypothesis, permit conclusions to be drawn, and thereby to develop or contribute to generalizable knowledge"—and defined *research* as "usually described in a formal protocol that sets forth an objective and a set of procedures designed to reach that objective." The commission declined the advice of some commentators to treat all medical innovations as research. Rather, it concluded that treatments and procedures that were novel and deviated from common practice ("innovative therapy") did not amount to research unless formally structured as a research project. However, because of concern that innovative therapies were being administered in an unsupervised way as medical practice, the commission concluded that "radical" or "major" innovations in therapy should be conducted as research, to establish their safety and efficacy.

These views were presented in a section of the Belmont Report called "Boundaries between Research and Practice," as follows:

> It is important to distinguish between biomedical and behavioral research, on the one hand, and the practice of accepted therapy on the other, in order to know what activities ought to undergo review for the protection of human subjects of research. The distinction between research and practice is blurred partly because both often occur together (as in research designed to evaluate a therapy) and partly because notable departures from standard practice are often called "experimental" when the terms "experimental" and "research" are not carefully defined.
>
> For the most part, the term "practice" refers to interventions that are designed solely to enhance the well-being of an individual patient or client and that have a reasonable expectation of success. The purpose of medical or behavioral practice is to provide diagnosis, preventive treatment or therapy to particular individuals. By contrast, the term "research" designates an activity designed to test an hypothesis, permit conclusions to be drawn, and thereby to develop or contribute to generalizable knowledge (expressed, for example, in theories, principles, and statements of relationships). Research is usually described in a formal protocol that sets forth an objective and a set of procedures designed to reach that objective.
>
> When a clinician departs in a significant way from standard or accepted practice, the innovation does not, in and of itself, constitute research. The fact that a procedure is "experimental," in the sense of new, untested or different, does not automatically place it in the category of research. Radically new procedures of this description should, however, be made the object of formal research at an early stage in order to determine whether they are safe and effective. Thus, it is the responsibility of medical practice committees, for example, to insist that a major innovation be incorporated into a formal research project.
>
> Research and practice may be carried on together when research is designed to evaluate the safety and efficacy of a therapy. This need not cause any confusion

regarding whether or not the activity requires review; the general rule is that if there is any element of research in an activity, that activity should undergo review for the protection of human subjects. (Belmont Report 1979)

Dr. Levine later wrote that novelty should not be the defining characteristic of research versus practice. Rather, it was whether the therapy had been validated as safe and effective (Levine 1986). He therefore favored use of the term *nonvalidated practices* for therapies that have not been tested sufficiently often or sufficiently well to predict safety and efficacy. Accepted therapies could also become "nonvalidated" if questions of efficacy and safety, like a newly discovered drug toxicity, arise at any point after initial validation. Levine wrote that all "nonvalidated practices" should be conducted as research but that the research should not interfere with basic medical practice objectives, whether therapeutic, diagnostic, or prophylactic. He pointed out that many therapies have not been validated in the strict sense, that he was not advocating, for instance, that the use of pediatric drugs (80% of which had not then been validated by research evidence) be reviewed by an IRB and subjected to formal research before being prescribed. He also acknowledged the difficulty of exercising judgment to determine what level of departure from accepted medical practice would trigger a requirement for administration under a research protocol.

Neither the statements included in the Belmont Report nor Levine's later comments settled the matter of how to distinguish medical practice from research, especially as it applied to innovations. One reason was that enough latitude had been left in the definitions to allow significant variation in how activity was classified. Another was the difficulty of following the general rule suggested in the Belmont Report of subjecting all "major" innovation to research. A third developed with the significant changes in medicine that occurred after the Belmont Report was published in the late 1970s.

Before the Belmont Report was published, U.S. physicians tended to practice singly or in small group practices, unless congregated in an academic institution. Decisions about the adoption of medical innovations were in the hands of the physicians, and, in that fee-for-service world with permissive insurance coverage, there were few barriers—and even a financial incentive—to use new technologies. Since then, physicians have tended to practice in larger groups and to see more patients; academic physicians have also become more entrepreneurial. But all physicians now work in an increasingly cost-conscious managed-care environment. It has become uncommon for third-party payers to cover nonvalidated treatments without cost-benefit and efficacy data. This requirement, coupled with an increase in private and public funding for medical research, caused the number of formal clinical research projects to escalate.

This escalation was accompanied by changes in the standards and the climate for research. Human research is no longer viewed as necessarily risky, nor are human subjects considered uniformly vulnerable. The doctor-patient relationship has changed from paternalistic to one in which the doctor's duty is often to respect and facilitate the patient's right to make autonomous medical decisions. Consequently, patients feel freer to make requests of their physicians; they often want access to the new treatments available in research programs and to the added medical care that sometimes comes with them. Patient advocacy groups energetically request research on products that may help their members; women want research projects to include them, so that the resulting health data will not apply only to men. Pediatricians have long demanded that more treatment research be conducted in children, despite the medical and legal risks.[3]

Increased human research activity has created a situation in which IRBs are regularly overwhelmed with requests to review and approve protocols. So much research is being conducted that independent for-profit entities called clinical research organizations (CROs) now exist to manage research trials, and there is a new profession, "research reviewer." Competition for research patients also now exists; medical centers and pharmaceutical companies vie for access to qualified research subjects. At the same time, research review and approval processes governed by IRBs have become more rigorous and time consuming (some say bureaucratic, rigid, and slow) and increasingly expensive. The result of these changes is that we are now experiencing a renewed reluctance by physicians to subject their medical innovations to research.

Ethical concerns about human research have also increased since the time of the Belmont Report. In 2002, in response to some high-profile human research deaths, the Department of Health and Human Services commissioned the Institute of Medicine (IOM) to study reports of various potential research problems, including conflicts of interest, inadequate safety monitoring, and insufficient communication to research subjects.[4] The resulting IOM report concluded that many changes were needed in the way studies were being conducted if they were to satisfy existing standards for the responsible conduct of research. These corrections included the accreditation of IRBs and the improvement of ethical review of protocols, access to information by subjects and monitors, informed consent, safety monitoring, and compensation for injured subjects (Federman, Hanna, and Rodriguez 2002). Reinforcing the requirements for the safe and ethical treatment of research subjects is surely a laudable goal, but, unfortunately, the added rigor has lessened physicians' interest in submitting innovative treatment modalities to an IRB.

As changes in the medical and research climates have continued, so have changes that more directly influence innovation and the divide between human research and medical practice. The pace and sophistication of medical innovation have both increased, as has the ability of new therapies to affect disease. Physicians have become more technologically adept and patient knowledge about and demand for access to new treatments has also increased. Levine's "nonvalidated practices" seem to have become more the norm than the exception—even in the case of medical products that are researched and heavily regulated. For instance, even though the FDA regulates the approval and marketing of drugs, physician prescribing is often either off-label or experimental. Thus, once a drug comes onto the market, its use is often for indications different from those in the research that led to its approval. In this sense, off-label use is experimental. In addition, knowledge about human and disease variability has expanded, and it is no longer assumed that FDA approval connotes general safety and efficacy for the approved indication. Now, physicians recognize that they do not know what to expect when a newly approved drug is used for patients who are infants, elderly, obese, pregnant, taking other drugs, or experiencing other diseases. These variations on the studied use of the drug may proceed as trial-and-error medical practice. Then, when physicians become convinced of efficacy, they often publish their findings on the drug's actions in specific populations. The situation is similar in surgery. One physician has described a contemporary tendency in surgical innovation that combines aspects of both clinical treatment and research but that proceeds as treatment, the results of which are published. Of this blended form of surgical innovations, he wrote that:

> 1) they [involve] a series of patients; 2) outcome measures are common clinical parameters, the type usually obtained during routine clinical follow up; 3) effectiveness is determined by comparison with historical controls; 4) formal written protocols do not exist; and 5) because these activities are viewed as clinical care, they are invisible to institutional review boards. Studies that show some potential may be presented at scientific meetings, reported in . . . peer-review journals, prepared for abstract, or submitted for publication as a "retrospective study," "pilot study," "case series," or "observational study." Although there is no collective title given to these types of studies, terms often used to describe their conceptual framework are informal research, hypothesis exploring data collection, preliminary clinical work, or informal data collection. (Margo 2001, p. 40)

The author's opinion was that most of this work was disguised research and that, to protect patients' right to informed consent, it should be treated as research. Others who have recently struggled with this issue have argued that, because the steady advance of medical knowledge causes medical practice to change continually, most medical therapies can be considered "nonvalidated." Although it seems counterintuitive, uncertainties about treatments often expand the more we learn about their effects. Because customary and accepted medical practice is less and less a static entity, what constitutes sufficient validation of safety and efficacy is often a moving target, even for treatments and devices that have been approved by regulatory agencies.

Thus, opinions about what constitutes the practice of medicine as opposed to research have continued to vary. Although sophisticated medical specialists sometimes believe that their practice creates unique conditions that make it difficult to follow the Belmont Report guidelines (Dosseter 1990; Frost 1998), most thinking on this topic has involved reiterations of the issues addressed by the Belmont Report commissioners.

The impact of recent changes on how medical innovation is being deployed is not yet clear. What is clear, however, is that the technological sophistication and pace of medical and surgical innovation will continue to increase. New technologies will remain costly and will consume an ever-increasing share of limited health care budgets. Some claim that the central challenge for modern health care organizations may become how to optimize medical technology management to foster the development and timely adoption of new technologies, procedures, and clinical practices that can deliver the best medical care and the highest patient satisfaction at the lowest cost. Whether this challenge can be met is open to debate. But in the future of a troubled health care system, the importance of medical innovation is destined to become even more prominent. That makes it essential, as well as opportune, to consider the processes of innovation and the ethical questions it raises.

CHAPTER TWO

The Modern History
of Human Research Ethics

Just as it is instructive to understand the history of medical practice innovations and the attempts to distinguish it from medical research, it is likewise helpful to be acquainted with the modern history of research on humans and how it led to the formalized ethics obligations of researchers and to the protections currently afforded to human subjects. Knowing this history enhances one's ability to make judgments about choices between medical practice innovation or research. Like the phases of medical practice innovations, the modern history of human research comprises a repeating cycle of innovation and advancement, controversial or abusive practices, and the development of either voluntary codes or laws and regulations to modify conduct.

It is an underappreciated fact that one of the first sets of modern laws requiring protection of human subjects of research was enacted in Germany before the Third Reich (Vollmann and Winau 1996a, 1996b). At the time, the governments in some countries, including the United States, were contemplating regulations to ensure the responsible conduct of research on humans (Jonsen 1998). Those beginnings had not yet borne fruit, most likely because physician control and autonomy in choosing how to conduct research was the established status quo. Germany's "Reich Circular of 1931" changed the situation when it set clear ethical standards that must be met to use humans in medical research. Under this law, which built on a 1900 directive from the Prussian minister for religious, educational, and medical affairs, the following requirements were set: consent must be obtained before a person could participate in research and this consent must be given in a clear and unmistakable manner; appropriate information about the research must be given to the potential subject; consent must be bona fide; the research design must be careful; and there must be special protections for vulnerable subjects. The motivation to pass this law came from the introduction of scientific and experimental methodology into clinical medicine in the nineteenth century. The increase in human research that followed (mostly using hospitalized patients) resulted in public disclosures that much of the research was done without the patients' consent and some of the experiments caused injury. A public outcry and debate ensued in Germany and elsewhere about whether the imperatives of scientific progress should outweigh the ethical treatment of human subjects.

That the 1931 German research law was not followed under the Third Reich has been attributed to the fact that some prominent German physicians had become adherents of using medicine to protect the genetic health of the German people. At the end of the nineteenth century, principles of racial hygiene arose that called for the protection of the German "germ plasm." Proponents recommended that the country meet this goal by preventing the breeding of "inferiors," the celibacy of the upper classes, and the appeals of feminists to limit reproduction. The Nazi tenet of the purity of the German race was in accord with these principles and practices. After Hitler signed a memo denying citizenship rights to certain groups of people deemed undesirable, laws were passed compelling those with genetic diseases to be sterilized, forbidding Jews to marry Aryans, and denying citizenship to and expelling Jews, homosexuals, Communists, Gypsies, and others. The characterization of these groups of people as inferiors led to their being used in the heinous experiments conducted by Nazi physicians like those who were later tried for their crimes at Nuremberg. Disclosures from these trials led to the establishment of the two most prominent human research codes of ethics, the Nuremberg Code (1947, written by the judges who tried the Nazi physicians) and the Declaration of Helsinki (1964, written by the World Medical Association and revised several times since). Both of these documents contain provisions common to the prior German laws, and they form the basis for all of the subsequently enacted international and domestic research ethics codes and regulations. (See Appendixes A and B of this volume.)

Neither the existence of the new international codes of ethics nor the protests against the unethical research that served as their genesis stopped human research abuses. Before World War I, groups such as the Anti-Vivisection Society had campaigned ardently in the United States to stop nonconsensual research and the use of the terminally ill and orphans in medical experiments. To no avail, these advocacy groups fought with the medical establishment and against the preva-

lent view that the authority of the physician governed decisions about what treatments were best for patients and what experiments would promote medical
progress. During World War II, the U.S. government sponsored war-related medical research programs, often in prisons, mental hospitals, and military camps,
and participation in these studies was deemed to be patriotic. After the Nuremberg doctors' trial, the influence of the new research ethics code was blunted by
the further intensification of medical research on behalf of the Cold War effort.

Starting in the 1940s and lasting almost thirty years in the United States,
dozens of government-sponsored studies were carried out to test reactions to radiation exposure (U.S. Department of Energy 1993). The primary reason for the
research was to determine the effects of radiation on soldiers and civilians in the
event of atomic war. While this research was under way, top level officials were
attempting to develop and communicate standards for the responsible conduct of
the research, but the process was inconsistent and standards were not disseminated or enforced. As a result, a significant number of the human studies were
performed without the understanding or consent of the subject patients. Examples of these studies included a Manhattan Project experiment in which hospitalized patients were injected with plutonium and other radioactive materials
without their consent. In another 1940s experiment, at Vanderbilt University,
820 pregnant women were given radioactive iron to study the effects on fetuses.
Evidence exists that informed consent was not obtained, and the children of these
women were later found to have a higher than normal cancer rate. In the 1950s
at Montefiore Hospital in New York City, a Jewish hospital with German Jewish
refugee physicians on staff, twelve cancer patients (ten of whom were terminally
ill) were injected with radioactive calcium and strontium-85 to measure the rate
at which radioactive substances were absorbed into human tissues. The patients
were not informed of the risks of exposure to radiation. Prisoners in Oregon from
1963 to 1971 had their testicles exposed to x-rays in an attempt to understand the
effects of radiation on the production and function of sperm. Subjects were com-
pensated for their participation and for each biopsy. All subjects who had not been
previously vasectomized agreed to undergo a vasectomy at the conclusion of the
study. All did so and received additional compensation for the procedure. These
subjects were not told of a risk of cancer from exposure to radiation.

Abuses in other medical research were also occurring during this time. For
example, in the 1960s at the Jewish Chronic Disease Hospital, live cancer cells
were injected into twenty-two elderly, debilitated patients to study the role of the
immune system in defending against cancer. No consent had been obtained. At
the Willowbrook State School in New York State, mentally impaired children were

infected with live hepatitis A virus in a search for ways to reduce the spread of fecal-borne infections. By all accounts, the children's parents were inadequately informed. Experiments on psychiatric patients also took place in the 1960s without the patients' consent. Presumably, the research physicians conducting these experiments were aware of the Nuremberg Code and the reasons for it. Yet, according to the Department of Energy report that revealed the existence of the radiation experiments, there seemed to be a view in the United States that the Nuremberg Code applied to barbarians such as the Nazis but not to ordinary physicians, especially those who felt that the research was justified by national security and Cold War considerations. Despite these views, revelations of ethically problematic research led the National Institutes of Health (NIH) to begin reviews of the research policies of its grantee medical research institutions. The reports from those reviews challenged the prevalent view that the judgment of the individual physician researcher was sufficient to assure that research was conducted in a responsible manner.

In 1966, awareness of ethical problems associated with human research grew when Harvard professor Henry Beecher began publishing descriptions of U.S. studies that failed to adhere to the Nuremberg Code (Beecher 1966a, 1966b). In these studies, Dr. Beecher revealed systematic violations of the rights of human subjects. Beecher disclosed in his references where these violations had taken place (many had occurred in prominent medical facilities), and the revelations initiated a series of events that resulted in a strengthening of research protections, including the American Medical Association's adoption of "Ethical Guidelines for Clinical Investigation by the AMA," and the alteration of the NIH's and the FDA's investigator guidelines to require superintendence by peers and evidence of informed consent in all human experiments. However, despite their abhorrence of the discovered research abuses, Beecher and many other research physicians did not favor outside control over medical experimentation. Rather, they preferred to rely in the integrity of the researcher who, informed of the problems, was expected to voluntarily conform to ethical research practices. This view was the product of their strong belief in the importance of medical research and in the unacceptability of conditions that would impede its progress. Beecher expressed this view in his book on the subject when he wrote that "the well-being, the health, even the actual or potential life of all human beings, born or unborn, depend upon the continuing experimentation in man. Proceed it must; proceed it will" (Beecher 1970).

In the 1970s, further disclosures of research abuses included the infamous Tuskegee syphilis study, conducted by the U.S. Public Health Service from 1932 to 1972 and stopped when it was disclosed in newspapers. The ethical violations in this study were numerous and included deceptive recruitment of 400 African American men with syphilis who were told they would receive "special free treatment," when the actual intent was to study the natural history of untreated syphilis. Penicillin was withheld from the subjects even after it had been shown to cure the disease. The rationale for the decision to withhold the medication was that these impoverished men would not have had access to penicillin anyway, so that continuing the study observations without it was unlikely to alter the medical fate of these men. In the words of one investigator, the study was important and the circumstances amounted to a "never-to-be-repeated opportunity" (Angell 1997, p. 847). Researchers even went so far as to claim that the data would be most helpful to people like the subjects, the rural poor with a high rate of untreated syphilis. Ironically, the investigators belatedly learned that the study data had become compromised because many of the subjects had been treated for syphilis by other doctors.

Human behavioral research also became a subject of ethics scrutiny. One notable example was the Stanford University prison study that took place in the 1970s when Professor Philip Zimbardo recruited and paid seventy college students to participate in a two-week study about prison life. Some students were designated as prisoners. They were "arrested" at their homes, booked at a real jail, then blindfolded and driven to a fake jail in the basement of a Stanford building. There, other students, who had been given the role of guards and instructed to maintain control without using physical violence, proceeded to use steadily increasingly coercive and aggressive tactics, humiliation, and dehumanization of the prisoners, to the point where stress reactions among the "prisoners" became unacceptable and some had to be released before the end of the study. Still, Zimbardo believed in the value of the study, which was designed to understand prison guards' behavior, and was initiated in the wake of a widely publicized prisoner death at San Quentin prison and of deadly retributions by guards at Attica prison following an inmate rebellion. Zimbardo believes that the study was ethical in that it followed current Stanford ethical guidelines and was carefully monitored. But, he said, it was also unethical "because people suffered and others were allowed to inflict pain and humiliation on their fellows over an extended period of time" (O'Toole 1997). The reports of such ethically controversial studies led commentators to ask a fundamental values question: When can a society condone exposing a few people to harm to benefit the many?

In response to revelations of abuses and to professional and lay commentary upon them, the 1970s became a time of research ethics activity in the federal government in the United States. In 1971, the Department of Health, Education, and Welfare produced guidelines on the protection of human subjects (which formalized the NIH guidelines) and led to the mandate that an institutional review board (IRB) review and approve all federally sponsored human research experiments before their commencement and periodically thereafter. IRBs were required to determine whether subjects would be placed at risk and, if risk was involved, whether (1) the risks to the subject were so outweighed by the sum of the benefit to the subject and the importance of the knowledge to be gained as to warrant a decision to allow the subject to accept these risks, (2) the rights and welfare of any such subjects would be adequately protected, (3) legally effective informed consent would be obtained by adequate and appropriate methods, (4) the conduct of the activity would be reviewed at timely intervals. In 1974, Congress passed the National Research Act and established the National Commission for the Protection of Human Subjects of Biomedical and Behavioral Research, which was to make recommendations about the basic ethical principles that should underlie the conduct of human research and to develop guidelines to assure that such research was conducted in accordance with those principles. This effort led to the publication in 1979 of the Belmont Report, which produced a set of ethical principles for human research and described the ways to implement those principles (i.e., informed consent, assessment of risks and benefits, equitable subject selection), including guides for research on human fetuses, children, prisoners, and recommendations on the functions of the IRBs.

The Belmont Report also set forth the distinctions between medical research and medical practice quoted in Chapter 1. The recommendations in the Belmont Report subsequently informed the 1981 President's Commission for the Study of Ethical Problems in Medicine and Biomedical and Behavioral Research, which developed what is now known as the Common Rule, endorsing the ethical principles articulated in the Belmont Report (*Code of Federal Regulations*). The Common Rule focuses on the requirements for IRB supervision of human research and for the informed consent of subjects. Other subparts of this regulation list rules that govern research on pregnant women, human fetuses and neonates, prisoners, and children. A description of the regulations is in Appendix C of this volume. Subsequently, the FDA changed its informed consent and IRB regulations to bring them into general conformity with the Common Rule. By 1991, the Common Rule had been adopted by almost all of the other U.S. government agencies that sponsor or conduct human research. Adherence to the Common Rule is not required of nonfederally funded research unless the research is performed at an institution whose research is subject to a multiple project assurance

(MPA), which, in essence, obliges the institution to apply the DHHS human subject protections to all of its human research (U.S. DHHS, Office for Human Research Protections). Over the years, many state governments have also adopted laws and regulations that control the conduct of human research.

The adoption of these formal research protections changed and regularized the conduct of human research in the United States. IRB review and requirements for informed and written consent and protection of vulnerable people became the norm. There was little doubt at the time that these protections would elevate the conduct of medical research. However, the requirements for IRB oversight and research protections did not anticipate the remarkable expansion in the prevalence, scope, and sophistication of human medical research. The volume of studies needing review began to strain the system's ability to impose, monitor, and enforce ethical requirements. And, as before, ethical lapses continued to be reported. In response, the government has been making further attempts to identify the scope of the problem. In the mid-1990s, an FDA study of IRBs revealed that 38 percent had deficiencies in their informed consent procedures. In 1996, a General Accounting Office study of 69 drug researchers, who had been issued enforcement letters by the FDA, revealed serious misconduct, including failure to obtain informed consent, forgery of subjects' signatures on informed consent forms, failure to inform patients that a drug was experimental, and fabrication of data to make subjects eligible for study (U.S. General Accounting Office 1996). In 1998, a DHHS inspector general's report reached the "troubling central conclusion" that the IRB system was in jeopardy. It noted, among many things, that some boards spent only a minute or two evaluating each complex clinical study (U.S. DHHS, Office of Inspector General 1998). Researchers began to complain that it took too long to obtain a review and approval of protocols and that the requirements for human subject protection were becoming burdensome. Throughout the 1990s, DHHS, through its Office for Protection from Research Risks (OPRR), investigated a series of research ethics and oversight violations of research institutions with MPAs.[1] (The DHHS Office for Protection from Research Risks is now the Office for Human Research Protections.)

The investigations resulted in the closing of research programs at multiple high-level research institutions and the imposition of other disciplinary actions. The investigated incidents included the suicide of a California research subject in a study of schizophrenia (the informed consent for which lacked adequate explanations of the risks either of the study medication or the alternative treatments available) and the death of a healthy 19-year-old student at the University of Rochester (resulting in the finding that researchers had failed to follow protocol requirements for the conduct of a medical procedure and limits on the use of anesthesia). Other research scandals that came to light during this time included a plastic surgery study at a New York hospital in which two different kinds of face lifts were performed on subjects, one on each side of the face, in a nonapproved study that did not inform the patients that they were participating in an experiment. That the study was not federally funded and not subject to the Common Rule did not blunt the criticism of it. In another incident, a Florida eye surgeon used his experimental cutting tool on sixty corneal transplant patients in a study that was not IRB approved and in which patients did not give informed consent for the use of the device (National Bioethics Advisory Commission 2001). These last two cases might qualify as instances in which the physician was at least ambivalent about whether the surgery was research or innovative medical practice. The physicians in both studies were disciplined.

In 1995, the National Bioethics Advisory Commission (NBAC) was formed by President Clinton to study important biomedical ethical issues, the first being the protection of the rights and welfare of human research subjects. In its report on this topic, *Ethical and Policy Issues in Research Involving Human Participants*, NBAC concluded that, although medical research was highly valuable, the system under which it was being conducted was flawed and in need of reform, because research subjects were inadequately protected, bureaucracy was excessive, research protection rules and the interpretation of them were confusing and conflicting, and the ability to respond to emerging areas of research was inadequate. NBAC recommended the creation of a new oversight system that was more responsive to these problems and that had more authority within the federal system for research oversight (National Bioethics Advisory Commission 2001). NBAC's reports coupled with continuing research investigations and enforcement actions led to extensive commentary in the medical literature and at conferences on the state of human research ethics. Some, like Professor Zimbardo, who had conducted the Stanford prison experiment (see above), told reporters that he believed that the pendulum had swung too far toward protecting research subjects at the expense of new knowledge that could help society (O'Toole 1997). However, the majority of the commentators held the belief that the continuous stream of violations meant that the human research system was broken. Shoring up this belief were two highly visible research ethics scandals in the early 2000s at two of the top research universities in the country.

The first case involved the death of Jesse Gelsinger, the 19-year-old mentioned above, from liver problems and multiple organ failure believed to be caused by a massive inflammatory reaction to his experimental treatment. Gelsinger had volunteered for a study to test the safety of a gene therapy vector intended to be used for ornithine transcarbamylase deficiency, a genetic condition of the liver that Gelsinger suffered from but in its mild form. Investigations revealed, among other violations, that (1) the information given to Gelsinger about the study was incomplete, (2) the researchers had not disclosed to the FDA or the study subjects that serious liver reactions had occurred in similar trials in animals, (3) some of the human subjects in the study had experienced liver enzyme elevations but that not all had been reported, (4) subjects were not monitored properly, and (5) some of the research subjects, including Gelsinger, did not fit the research protocol enrollment requirements. As a result of these violations, the gene therapy research program, which was considered to be the best in the nation, was shut down by the FDA, federal legal action against the university and the researchers resulted in fines and research restrictions, a lawsuit was brought by Gelsinger's family, and the entire field of gene therapy research suffered a serious setback (Nelson and Weiss 1999; Marshall 2000). The second major scandal involved the death of Ellen Roche, a healthy 24-year-old lab technician at Johns Hopkins University. Roche volunteered to take part in a study intended to enhance the understanding of the causes of asthma. She was administered the inhaled drug hexamethonium which led to her death from lung failure after several weeks in an intensive care unit. Investigations revealed that the researchers who conducted the experiment and the IRB that approved it had failed to take adequate precautions to protect the study's research subjects. The principal investigator had overlooked some prior research concluding that hexamethonium might be toxic to the lung, and the subjects were not told that the substance might be harmful or that it was not approved by the FDA. In addition, Roche, who was the third subject in the trial, was not told (nor was the IRB) that the first subject had developed a cough and shortness of breath that lasted a week after inhaling the drug (Kolata 2001). The federal Office of Human Research Protection (which was the more authoritative office recommended by NBAC) also harshly criticized the Johns Hopkins system for reviewing experiments and suspended most federally funded experiments at Hopkins and several affiliated institutions, almost 2,000 studies, until additional review could be completed on them.

News coverage of these events was extensive and led investigative reporters to uncover more questionable studies and an uneven application of federal research standards (Kaplan and Brownlee 1999). This kind of coverage has led to fears that the public would begin to lose trust in the American medical research endeavor. The concern was succinctly expressed by Ezekiel Emanuel, from the Department of Clinical Bioethics at the NIH. Dr. Emanuel's remarks were presented to NBAC's successor, the President's Council on Bioethics, at its meeting in September 2002.

> Today, almost no one is happy with the process of protecting human participants in clinical research. Clinical investigators are frustrated with the review process, which seems bureaucratic and inefficient, burdening them with minor details rather than helping them ensure participants' safety. IRB members feel overworked, baffled by ambiguous regulations, fearful of federal audits, and anxious about calls for accreditation of uncertain benefit. Federal regulators are aggravated by the limited scope of their authority and variable adherence to regulations, and worried about criticism from Congress and the public for inaction in the face of mounting harms to research participants. Commercial sponsors of clinical research see the system as time consuming, repetitive, and inefficient, with delays costing millions of dollars. Foreign researchers and governments often view the imposition of U.S. regulations as culturally insensitive and even imperialistic. The public finds each death during a research study and each new case of allegedly unethical practices worrisome and indicative that the system is broken. (Quoted in Wood, Grady, and Emanuel 2002)

With concerns such as these, it is easy to see how some physicians prefer to introduce their medical innovations as clinical practice if they can. The history of modern medical research also highlights the fact that the same tensions exist among the imperatives of medical progress, physician authority, and patient protection and autonomy in medical research as in clinical practice. How any changes in federal standards for either will influence the deployment choice and the tensions remains to be seen.

CHAPTER THREE

Innovation in the Off-Label
Use of Drugs

THE BACKGROUND

Innovation in drug therapy often occurs in the unregulated "off-label" use of drugs. The term *off-label* comes from the FDA's regulation of what uses a drug is approved for and what claims a pharmaceutical company is allowed make about any approved drug. Because all of this information is included in the drug's labeling, using a drug for an unapproved purpose has come to be called "off-label use." Central to the FDA's marketing approval process is the approval of a drug's labeling, which technically includes the label affixed to the drug's container, a package insert that accompanies the drug and contains full information about its effects, and certain advertising. The label information, whether on the container, on the package insert, or in any advertising or promotion, is limited to describing the drug's use *only* for the approved doses and routes of administration for the approved medical condition. The use of a drug under circumstances not included in the labeling is considered to be a nonapproved, or off-label, use.

Pharmaceutical companies are forbidden by law to promote off-label drug use unless they follow narrow "safe harbor" conditions.[1] However, because the FDA does not regulate the practice of medicine, physicians may prescribe a drug for an off-label use if it seems reasonable or appropriate. Physicians possess a largely unfettered professional prerogative to use approved drugs for any medically reasonable purpose, and a significant amount of off-label drug use is introduced as medical practice innovation and not as research. Off-label use can start when a physician guesses, based on what is known about a drug and/or a disease, that a drug might also be useful for another medical condition. Physicians also obtain information about off-label use from the medical literature (physicians sometimes write case reports of nonapproved uses) and from colleagues, who often relate their experiences with off-label use at professional meetings.

It is easiest to explain off-label use of drugs with an example. One involved the use of theophylline for patients with a lung condition called chronic obstructive pulmonary disease (COPD), the major symptom of which is shortness of breath. Theophylline was known to relax and dilate the airways in patients with asthma and was approved for use in patients with that condition. The drug was also widely used for decades in adults with nonasthmatic COPD. Even though there was no pharmacologic reason to believe that the drug would work and it was known that the drug could be quite toxic, many physicians prescribed theophylline for COPD because many patients had reported that it helped their breathing. Finally, research was conducted which showed that, at sufficient blood levels, the drug improved lung function compared with placebo treatment and was tolerable (Eaton et al. 1980). During the years that theophylline was being prescribed for COPD without any research data to support its use, many patients undoubtedly benefited.

This example explains why many physicians would object if the FDA interfered with their professional judgment to use an approved drug for an unapproved purpose. Regulation, they say, would stifle the significant advances that can be made with drug treatments. Conversely, proponents of regulation believe that unresearched off-label drug use is risky and needs oversight, because no research has advised the physician about whether a drug works consistently. Also, off-label drug use, even if widespread, does not serve to inform the medical community about the full consequences of the use—what conditions maximize its benefit and minimize its toxicity. Only systematic and controlled research can accomplish that goal, they argue. In the theophylline example, research showed doctors that doses of the drug below certain levels produced no clinically significant improvements in lung function while subjecting the patient to the risk of toxicity. Finally, some who would change the status quo are troubled by the fact that most patients are not told by their physicians that the drug they have been prescribed has not been approved for use in their condition (Beck and Azari 1997; Salbu 1999; Zindrick 2000).

If research and regulation do not govern the off-label use of drugs, what does? Physicians are held to the "standard of care" within the medical community. Legally, the standard of care is determined by what expert physicians will testify is considered generally accepted practice by other physicians practicing in the same area of medicine. However, the standard of care is an ever-evolving bench-mark; and many times, physicians will disagree about where permitted bound-aries lie. What constitutes accepted practice consequently can be fairly broad. Holding physicians to the standard of care is thus dependent upon challenges of suspect practice. Any challenges to an individual physician's professional behav-ior will come from hospital credentialing and peer review committees, from state physician licensing agencies, or in the courtroom through medical malpractice litigation. Reviews under these systems usually take place only after patients have been injured or when someone, usually a patient, complains about what the doc-tor has done. The outcome of such a complaint depends on the reasonableness of the doctor's judgment. Certainly, physicians can be held liable for negligence or put their license at risk if their off-label applications are sufficiently careless, imprudent, or otherwise unprofessional, but they also risk liability if they fail to provide appropriate treatment solely because it involves the off-label use of a drug (Blum 2002).

Whether or not a patient benefits or is harmed by off-label drug use depends on a number of factors. These include the skill of the physician, how closely a pa-tient is monitored, and how much data exist to support the safety and effective-ness of the off-label use. If a physician is prompted to prescribe off-label for a pa-tient based on limited evidence, such as a few case reports in the literature, it may not be apparent that the patient in the office is different in some relevant way from the patients described in the literature. And sometimes this difference can cause the patient to react badly to the drug. On the other hand, as with the theo-phylline example above, many off-label uses have become the standard of care without the data from carefully controlled research, because of a gradual accu-mulation of a significant number of informal reports of successful use. Any pe-diatrician or gerontologist will point out that off-label prescribing occurs in part because most researchers are reluctant to enroll patients at the extremes of age in drug trials. It is also true that many physicians have come to believe that much of the research required by the FDA to support the marketing of a drug is unhelp-ful in the general practice of medicine. Studies performed for drug approval pur-poses often enroll study subjects who are more compliant, younger and healthier, have milder forms of the study disease, take fewer other drugs, have fewer con-current diseases, and take the drug for shorter periods of time than do the popu-lation of patients who ultimately receive the new drug. Therefore, practicing physicians frequently must prescribe without the guidance of controlled study data that relate specifically to their patient population. "What makes off-label pre-scribing much different from that?" they ask.

Given this state of affairs, it is not surprising that off-label drug prescribing is extensive. According to the U.S. General Accounting Office (1996), a number of studies from the early to mid-1990s documented that:

- 56 percent of cancer patients have been given off-label drug treatments and 33 percent of all cancer treatment prescriptions are off-label,
- 81 percent of AIDS patients received at least one drug off-label and 40 percent of all reported drug treatment in AIDS patients was off-label, and
- nearly all pediatric patients are prescribed drugs off-label, because many drugs are not tested for use in children.

Medical history is full of examples in which fortuitous discoveries led to the widespread use of a drug off-label and then to adoption of the new use as the standard of care. Amantadine is a well-known example. This medication was originally developed for the treatment of Parkinson disease. Physicians began noticing that Parkinson patients receiving amantadine, even those living in nursing homes, were not getting influenza. It is now an accepted anti-influenza medication. Dilantin, an antiseizure medicine, was first used to control peripheral neuropathy (numbness and tingling) in patients with diabetes; and minoxidil, originally an antihypertension drug, turned out also to stimulate hair growth and became the most widely prescribed drug (trade named Rogaine) for male pattern baldness. One of the most impressive off-label uses of drugs occurred early in the AIDS crisis, when the lives of thousands of patients were saved by the off-label use of various mixtures of antiretroviral and anti-infective drugs. In addition, any fairly nontoxic drug that also causes weight loss is invariably prescribed for obese patients. There are also plenty of examples in which off-label drug use did not pan out, such as when research showed that the weight loss seen in the early weeks of treatment with the antidepressant Prozac reversed after a few months. Other times, an off-label use is abandoned when physicians learn from experience—in their own practice or that of others—that it leads to unacceptable side effects. This is what happened when the diet drug combination called fen-phen (from fenfluramine and phentermine) was found to cause potentially lethal heart and lung damage. Nearly six million people took the drug combination before it was withdrawn from the market. Subsequently, tens of thousands of lawsuits were filed against the physicians who prescribed the drugs and the companies that sold them (Brosgart et al. 1996; Wangsness 2000).

The examples above show that, whether or not a drug is researched before use, patients can experience both benefit and harm. Therefore, whether off-label drug prescribing is beneficial or not, harmful or not, is often not the point. Rather, the conflict centers on which pathway to establishment of use is better, that is, whether medical knowledge is advanced and patients benefit more from drugs that are researched and regulated or from drug use that comes about through the practice of medicine (Flannery 1986; Serradell and Rucker 1990). Two quotes exemplify the debate.

[Human research] field trials are indispensable. They will continue to be an ordeal. They lack glamour, they strain our resources and patience, and they protract the moment of truth to excruciating limits. Still, they are among the most challenging of our skills. I have no doubt that when the problem is well chosen, the study is appropriately designed, and that when all the populations concerned are made aware of the route and goal, the reward can be commensurate with the effort. If, in major medical dilemmas, the alternative is to pay the cost of perpetual uncertainty, have we really any choice? (Frederickson 1968, p. 992)

Whatever costs, risks, or other disadvantages that might be associated with off-label prescription of drugs, two facts appear to be indisputable. First, some of the most effective drug treatments in existence today are off-label treatments. . . . Second, off-label prescription creates unique opportunities to witness the effects of new applications over the widest possible population and during the shortest possible period. Unfettered access to an entire population of patients provides an unrestricted, admittedly informal laboratory, thereby hastening medical advances. The costs and benefits of combination treatments will be revealed more quickly among the universe of patients than among a small sample of patients, and by a wide array of doctors rather than a handful of scientific investigators. Off-label prescription thus maximizes information and increases the speed with which it is amassed. Likewise, it multiplies the number of minds that will look at the information, apply different perspectives, and develop hypotheses, theories, and principles regarding a new treatment. The logical result of these dynamics should be to propel the state of the art of medical practice. (Salbu 1999, p. 218)

THE CASE STUDY

MegaPharm, Incorporated, has developed a drug that appears to be very effective in treating a certain rare subset of adult-onset (type 2) diabetes. The drug has been approved for that narrow indication by the FDA following a large-scale Phase III trial in one thousand patients. Previously, this form of type 2 diabetes was particularly resistant to treatment, and the new drug offers hope to the approximately 300,000 U.S. patients with this disease, many of whom develop serious complications, including heart attack and stroke, kidney failure, blindness, or vascular damage to the feet and legs that requires amputation. The drug was approved rapidly, under "fast track" and priority review conditions, because it was targeted at a serious unmet medical need and because the study data indicated that the drug was both safe and effective for lowering blood sugar in the study population.

The Professor and the Pharma

Professor Leptinski is an endocrinologist at a leading medical college and was the lead investigator on the diabetes drug trials. He and MegaPharm have been lauded for their research work, which led to the marketing of a badly needed drug. This research was not the first time that Dr. L had worked with MegaPharm. He had been a long-time consultant, and his drug studies on behalf of the company have always been first rate and reliable. His drug research has been published in prestigious medical journals. Theirs has been a successful collaboration and, as a consequence, a significant portion of Dr. L's research funding comes from MegaPharm. When Dr. L was involved in the diabetes drug trials, he noted that some of the participants in the trial reported, among other side effects of the drug, that they experienced weight loss and "lost appetite." These problems were listed as side effects on the drug's labeling, but Dr. L saw them as an opportunity because he guessed that the drug might be effective for weight loss.

Dr. Leptinski knows that there is a strong need for an effective and safe weight loss drug in the United States because in the last two decades, the incidence of obesity among adults and children has risen nearly 50 percent. As defined by federal standards, approximately 23 percent of adults and 11 percent of children are considered obese. The impact of obesity is enormous. According to the surgeon general, about 300,000 U.S. deaths each year are associated with obesity and overweight (approaching the 400,000 deaths a year associated with cigarette smoking). The total direct and indirect costs attributed to overweight and obesity amounted to $117 billion in the year 2000. If the new diabetes drug could also be used to treat obesity, tremendous health and health cost benefits could be achieved. Dr. L pursued this possibility in studies using an animal model, with very encouraging results. He then began lobbying MegaPharm to undertake the necessary R&D program to gain approval for this broader indication. He thought that MegaPharm would leap at the chance to study the drug's weight-loss potential because the market for the relatively rare diabetic disease for which the drug was approved was small.

However, because of the typical commitment of six to eight years and hundreds of millions of dollars to conduct clinical drug research and gain FDA approval, the company is reluctant to commit. Too many of the promising new molecules being developed for obesity treatment have failed in clinical trials, indicating to MegaPharm that not enough is known about the underlying physiology and biochemical influences of weight control to reliably develop a safe and effective drug. An additional deterrent is that antiobesity drugs, such as the notorious fen-phen combination, have garnered a bad reputation because they seem prone to causing severe side effects that prompt litigation against the manufacturer. Despite the fact that the antiobesity drug market could be huge (a breakthrough product in this market could net the company several billion dollars in annual sales), MegaPharm decides that its interests would be better served by staying out of the weight-loss market. If physicians choose to treat obesity with the drug, so be it. Provided that the company refrains from promoting the drug for this purpose, the added sales attributable to the off-label use will benefit the company but the responsibility for the drug's use in obesity will lie solely with the prescribing physicians.

1. Who has conflicts of interest in this scenario, and how do these conflicts play out?
2. Are there any ethical concerns about a pharmaceutical company's passively accepting the financial rewards of an off-label market?
3. Is the off-label prescribing of this drug the equivalent of experimental treatment, and should it be treated as such? Would it be feasible to subject all new uses of approved drugs to clinical studies before prescribing is allowed? Or should the decisions about off-label drug prescription be left to the medical professionals?

Dr. Leptinski Prescribes Off-Label

Undeterred, and convinced that the diabetes drug holds promise for weight reduction, Dr. L begins prescribing the drug off-label for clinically obese nondiabetic patients. Although he knows that the drug has the potential to cause significant side effects, Dr. L believes that the risks are reasonable, given the serious medical conditions and social problems attributable to obesity. This treatment also seems medically justifiable, because Dr. L suspects that the drug's side effects are primarily linked to the diabetic condition and that nondiabetic patients the risks to be lower. In addition, Dr. L hopes that if he is successful with his obese patients, that will prompt MegaPharm to support official clinical trials and seek FDA approval for the additional use. What he has not foreseen is that his clinic becomes known as a place to obtain diet pills, and, increasingly, patients who are overweight but not clinically obese begin to seek appointments and prescriptions from him. The demands increase after Dr. L reports his initial patient results (which he calls "promising") at a medical conference and some weight loss websites begin extolling the virtues of the drug.

General demand for the drug grows, and soon many physicians are prescribing the drug for weight loss, in both adults and children. As more medical journal articles (some of which are peer-reviewed and show that the drug is safer than amphetaminelike drugs) describe the drug's value for this unapproved use, the off-label prescriptions eventually account for more than 60 percent of the sales of the drug, significantly increasing MegaPharm's revenues. Some physicians, however, begin to voice the opinion that the unknown risks of the drug do not justify prescribing it to healthy overweight people. These physicians begin to refuse to prescribe the drug for any overweight patient who isn't morbidly obese. However, patients who are denied prescriptions by one physician always seem to find another who will prescribe. In addition, some patients who are adept at obtaining prescriptions willingly share them with friends.

4. What does this case suggest about the consequences of Dr. L's taking the "individual innovator" route rather than the more formal research route?
5. What disclosure obligations does Dr. L have in prescribing the new drug for obesity?
6. Should Dr. L limit his off-label prescribing of the drug to patients with the most severe forms of weight problems? How should he decide what the reasonable cut-offs are? How should patient demand figure into his decision?
7. Are additional professional practice laws needed to ensure responsible off-label prescribing?
8. Should drug manufacturers take any responsibility for the off-label use and prescription of their drug products?

MegaPharm Promotes

MegaPharm is impressed with the success of the off-label prescribing of this drug and becomes convinced of the benefits for obese patients. In addition, company managers are concerned about the increasingly frequent misconceptions about the drug found in both lay and professional publications and on weight loss web sites and chat rooms. Some of this information touts the benefits of the drug in overly optimistic terms and, likewise, some of the purported harms are exaggerated. Deciding it would be in the company's best interest, MegaPharm launches an off-label campaign and studies for the use of the drug in obesity. The purpose of the campaign is to foster responsible prescribing and to provide physicians with accurate information, so that they can better inform obese patients of the risks and benefits of the drug. MegaPharm also hopes that the campaign will increase sales and prompt third-party payers to cover the drug for this use. Mindful of the "safe harbor" provisions of FDAMA, the company is determined to stay within the bounds of the restrictions but knows that these are relatively uncharted waters. It is therefore difficult to know how the FDA, the medical professionals, and patients will respond to this campaign.

9. What are the benefits and risks of off-label drug prescribing and promotion? Should physicians be entitled to information from the manufacturer about off-label uses? Are there controls that can be implemented (by the FDA or the medical profession or the courts) that can maximize the benefit and minimize the harm of these activities?

Is the Drug Too Toxic?

Inevitably, as the number of patients taking the drug grows and the duration of use extends beyond the time studied in the original Phase III trials, reports of side effects begin to appear. At first, it is unclear whether the problems are caused by the underlying diseases of the patients or other drugs they are taking, or by the MegaPharm drug. For both the diabetic and the overweight patient populations, the side effects are generally those that were reported during the clinical trials of the drug. However, the company and the FDA begin to receive reports that some of the side effects are more severe than expected, specifically those related to the liver. These reports indicate a strong possibility of a causal link between the drug and liver problems. The FDA asks and the company agrees to place a "black box" on the drug labeling warning physicians to monitor for hepatic toxicity. When the reports of liver toxicity persist and the numbers of deaths and liver transplants reach 20 and 6, respectively, evenly divided between diabetic patients and nondiabetic obese patients, some physicians and patient advocacy groups begin lobbying to have the drug withdrawn from the market.[2] The spokesperson for one patient advocacy group complains that "peer review simply isn't as rigorous as traditional FDA-mandated clinical trials. Off-label use puts increased numbers of Americans at risk." On the other hand, the drug has its proponents, among them physicians who believe that the adverse reaction rate is no higher than that of a number of other highly useful drugs. What is needed, they say, is more careful monitoring.

The most vociferous support for the drug comes from the patients who had lost significant amounts of weight while taking it. One woman told a news reporter, "I would half-kill to stay on it. When I was fat, I hated myself. I knew my health was awful. I'm pretty sure it's why my husband left me. But if something else came along that would control my weight in the same way, I'd jump to it in a second, because I don't want to risk liver problems. But I also don't want to take any of those speed drugs either. I got hooked on them, they made my heart race, and I ignored my kids when I was on them. Then I lost fen-phen. So, as long as this new drug is still available, I'm taking it."

10. Current adverse drug reaction reporting is voluntary for physicians. Should more be done to monitor the off-label use of new drugs and assure reporting of side effects?

11. If this drug is recalled, whose responsibility should it be to address the complaints of patients (both diabetic and obese) who will be deprived of what they consider a vitally important drug?

Innovative Surgery

THE BACKGROUND

Innovations in the way surgeries are performed often occur with little or no advance oversight. If supervision is present, it is most likely done by medical-credentialing or peer review staff, who aim to assure that physicians are sufficiently skilled to perform a particular surgery at that hospital, or by the FDA if there is an innovative device involved, for the FDA tries to assure that surgical devices are safe and effective for their intended use. However, medical staffs do not often ask surgeons to be recredentialed when they alter a surgery they have privileges to perform, and the FDA does not regulate the manner in which surgeons use approved surgical devices. This means that, in a practice akin to off-label drug use, surgeons can use approved devices in novel ways without FDA oversight. More than other kinds of medical practice, innovative surgical techniques raise the issue of the variation in skill levels among physicians and the impact that has on deciding whether innovation should be deployed as surgical practice or research. The fact that surgeries are less amenable to evaluation by randomized controlled clinical trials often colors that choice.

An illustrative example of how surgical innovation occurs is what has become known as closed-chest, beating-heart cardiovascular surgery. In an article on the history of the development of cardiovascular surgery, pioneering surgeons Denton Cooley and Bud Frazier (Cooley and Frazier 2000) described their amazement at how fast the field had developed since it began in World War II. As happens in any war, battle conditions forced field surgeons to adopt novel techniques.

One of these surgeons, Dwight Harken, was praised for his courage in attempting the first surgical manipulations of the heart, something previously thought to be uniformly fatal. During World War II, more than one hundred soldiers survived the removal of shrapnel from their heart, and the specialty of cardiovascular surgery was born. Over the years since then, various problems had to be solved for the practice to advance. The first was to develop a way to interrupt blood flow during an intracardiac operation. Hypothermia was one of the early methods tried, either by placing patients in a tub of ice water or by cooling them with ice packs. If a patient's temperature could be lowered to about 26°C, blood flow to the heart could be interrupted and the heart stilled, and the patient could survive if the surgical repair could be accomplished within ten minutes. If the blood flow was stopped for any longer, brain damage was a certainty. As can be imagined, many patients did not survive these early surgeries, because of mishaps or air embolisms that infarcted the heart, brain, or lungs, or because the heart defect was too complicated to repair in the time required. To address some of these problems, John Gibbon worked for more than ten years to design a device that would provide for oxygenation and circulation of blood during open-heart surgery. He invented what has come to be called a cardiopulmonary bypass machine. It was first used in 1953 on four patients with congenital heart disease. Only one patient survived. Although Gibbon himself never again attempted open-heart surgery with his machine, others did, and the innovations continued.

Open-heart surgery on a stilled heart (a state now achieved with drugs) using a cardiopulmonary bypass machine eventually produced good results and achieved widespread acceptance. However, surgeons discovered that the cardiopulmonary bypass aspect of these surgeries was causing morbidity and death from systemic inflammatory reactions, blood-clotting disorders, impairment of brain function, and/or damage to major organs. In addition, splitting the sternum and spreading the rib cage to gain access to the heart caused significant morbidity (e.g., pain, infection, prolonged hospital stays, and recoveries with subsequent disabilities). So far, little has been accomplished to ameliorate the bypass machine problems, but surgeons have been able to eliminate the need to open the chest by developing radically new "minimally invasive" (sometimes also called "closed-chest" or "endoscopic") techniques. These surgeries are accomplished with the use of new microminiaturized surgical tools and endoscopic and video imaging technologies that have given surgeons the ability to operate without directly touching or seeing the organ on which they are working. Using specialized instruments inserted through the chest wall via small incisions, surgeons view the operative site on a monitor connected to a mini-camera inserted through another small inci-

sion in the chest wall. Although the new techniques are difficult to learn and surgeons still have to contend with the bypass machine problems, minimally invasive cardiac surgery offers the benefit of less trauma and shortened recovery time
with fewer postsurgical complications. It took until the middle to late 1990s to
develop these new techniques and tools for general cardiac surgical use, and by
that time the procedural and technological developments had generated both detractors and supporters within the surgical community.

Two of the detractors, Drs. Bonchek and Ullyot, had come to view open-chest
surgery using a cardiopulmonary bypass machine as the standard procedure for
repair of clogged coronary blood vessels, because of the procedure's widespread
use, its successful and reproducible outcomes, and the cost savings from the low
incidence of complications and less need for repeat vascularizations. In addition,
this was a teachable procedure, meaning that reasonably skilled cardiovascular
surgeons could, in a reasonable amount of time, become adept at performing the
operation. Bonchek and Ullyot deplored the rush to adopt the new minimally invasive techniques, claiming that it was too difficult for a surgeon to move from
being able to look directly at the heart being manipulated to an indirect approach
of maneuvering the surgical instruments while looking at a monitor suspended
over the operating table. Because of the difficulty of the technique, operative results were not reproducible from surgeon to surgeon, learning curves varied, and
patients suffered as a result. They concluded that just because a procedure could
be done did not mean that it should be done, and they then modified the axiom
further by stating that just because a procedure could be done by some surgeons
did not mean that it should be done by all surgeons (Bonchek and Ullyot 1998).
None other than the intrepid surgical pioneer Denton Cooley admitted that minimally invasive surgery could "challenge even the deftest of hands and may subject the patient to added risk" (Cooley and Frazier 2000, p. 92).

Other surgeons encouraged the adoption of noninvasive techniques. According to Mack et al. (1999, p. 1406), "For our specialty [cardiac surgery] to survive
and flourish in these rapidly changing times, we must have the courage to em-
brace the change and continually reinvent ourselves and our practices. Only our
ability to evolve will guarantee our survival. We must not become stagnant by the
inertia of our past success and fail to grasp the opportunity of change." Such enthusiasm, combined with patient demand accompanied by support from the medical device industry, drove the application of minimally invasive surgical techniques in cardiothoracic and other surgical specialties. The surgeons skilled at
minimally invasive techniques welcomed both the patient benefits and the competitive advantages the new skills gave them over surgeons using older techniques.

In the middle of the debate about minimally invasive procedures were surgeons who seemed to think that forging ahead was so embedded in the nature of
a surgeon that it was useless to debate whether they should. Among the histori-
cal accounts of the tenacity with which some surgeons pursue innovation is the
incident involving a German surgeon, Werner Forssmann, who was perfecting
the heart-catheterization procedure on animals and cadavers. He then asked two
surgical colleagues to assist him as he attempted to perform the first procedure
on a human—himself. Both surgeons refused, so he inserted the catheter into
his antecubital vein and threaded it to his heart unaided. He then walked to the
radiology department, where an x-ray confirmed the catheter placement in his
right atrium. Although he was criticized for this and fired from the hospital, his
"courage" in this regard was cited when he was awarded the Nobel Prize in Medicine in 1956 for his work in developing the new procedure. This account is described in the book *King of Hearts* (Miller 2000), as was the yet more dramatic
story of how Charles P. Bailey pioneered cardiac valve surgery (Weisse 2005).

In the late 1940s, there were no treatments that would prevent death in patients with valvular heart disease. Charles P. Bailey, of the Hahnemann Medical
College in Philadelphia, was determined to find a way to surgically correct one
form of this disease, mitral valve stenosis, a condition that had killed his father.
He had performed what he thought was a sufficient number of procedures on
dogs and human cadavers, with good results, and he performed his first procedure on a live person in 1945, on a 37-year-old man. The patient died on the operating table of massive bleeding. The fact that no surgeon until then had actually placed a finger inside of the heart of a living patient, coupled with Bailey's
reputation as an especially aggressive surgeon, led his colleagues to caution him
to stop his pursuit. Bailey was not deterred, however, and operated on his second
patient, a 29-year-old woman, who died two days after the surgery. At that point,
Bailey was told that he could no longer perform the operation at Hahnemann.
The chief of cardiology reportedly said that he had a Christian duty to prevent
Bailey from performing this "homicidal" procedure. Bailey is said to have replied
that it was *his* Christian duty to perfect the operation, because nothing was worse
than what mitral valve stenosis does to people. To circumvent the Hahnemann
restriction, Bailey scheduled his third mitral valve surgery at a hospital across the
state line in Delaware. This patient died on his fifth postoperative day from an
overdose of anticoagulant medication and fluids. Bailey was then told he could
no longer perform the procedure in the Delaware hospital. Afraid that he would
be permanently stopped, but still undeterred and convinced that the procedure

should work with more experience, Bailey did another end run. He scheduled two patients at two different Philadelphia hospitals on the same day, one at 8 A.M. and the second at 2 P.M. He figured that, if the first patient died in the operating room, word of the death would not reach the second hospital across town in time to prevent the second case from proceeding. The first patient did die during the surgery. The patient scheduled for 2 P.M. was a 24-year-old mother whose doctor had tried to dissuade her from having the operation. In her case, Bailey tried a new approach and a new instrument, and the woman survived. Ten days later, she traveled with Bailey to Chicago, where she was presented at the American College of Chest Physicians meeting as having had the first successful mitral valve surgery. The woman went on to have two more children, and she died thirty-eight years later of heart and lung failure probably caused by her cigarette smoking. Mitral valve surgery has since become life saving for untold numbers of patients.

Harvard surgeon Atul Gawande confirms that the fearlessness of surgeons in the face of uncertainty still exists:

> There is a saying about surgeons, meant as a reproof: "Sometimes wrong; never in doubt." But this seemed to me their strength. Every day, surgeons are faced with uncertainties. Information is inadequate; the science is ambiguous; one's knowledge and abilities are never perfect. Even with the simplest operation, it cannot be taken for granted that a patient will come through better off—or even alive. Standing at the table my first time [as a surgical intern], I wondered how the surgeon knew he would do this patient good, that all the steps would go as planned, that bleeding would be controlled and infection would not take hold and organs would not be injured. He didn't, of course. But he still cut. (Gawande 2002, pp. 15–16)

The cardiac surgeons who were attempting to develop minimally invasive surgery in the 1990s were most likely aware of their fearless predecessors Forssmann and Bailey, and advocates of the innovations came from that mold. Yet, there have also always been surgeons more inclined to caution, who want innovation to be guided by evidence. In the case of the new minimally invasive cardiac surgery, these surgeons wanted to know whether the patients' benefits were theoretical or real. But, the answer to the question depended on both the inherent qualities of the procedure and the skills of the surgeon involved. Any study addressing whether the improvements were "real" as opposed to only theoretical would have to ensure that all surgeons in the study used the same technique, were equally skilled, and that their patients were in the same category of risk. Surgical skill is difficult to assess, given that surgery is performed by a team, consisting of surgeons, anesthesiologists, nurses, and technicians. Patient risk category is also difficult to quantify because many of a patient's surgical risks are not evident until the surgery has revealed all of the internal pathology. These difficulties allowed the debates about the benefits and risks of open- versus closed-chest techniques to persist. In the meantime, surgeons were still attempting to address the adverse reactions associated with the use of cardiac bypass machines. Some were attempting to avoid the risks by developing surgical techniques that would do away with the machines altogether.

While the debates and the innovations continued, a dialogue arose in the surgical literature about the impact of surgical innovations on patients. In one paper (Bunch and Dvonch 2000), the authors noted that "innovation" could be the middle name of most orthopedic surgeons but that much innovation occurs without the consent of the patient. The authors stated that "the problem is how to think about innovation so to allow and encourage it and yet to protect the patient from the exploitation of being an 'experimental animal' " (p. 44). The question at the heart of this dilemma is what the patient should be told: That I want to cure you? That I haven't done many of these procedures? That I have failed x number of times? That I want to develop my skills? That I want to learn new information? That I hold the patent on the instruments I will use? In answering questions about the surgeon's disclosure duties, there seemed to be no consensus about what differentiated surgical research from innovative surgical care. New and highly risky surgery could be either. The absence of a research hypothesis and written protocol did not alone distinguish one from the other (Margo 2001). If, as required in most states, patients have the right to be told of the risks and benefits of a proposed medical treatment or surgery and of all reasonable alternatives, is this amount of disclosure enough when it comes to innovative surgery? Should the surgeon's motives also be disclosed? Should patients be told that their surgeon has performed the procedure only ten times before? that other surgeons are better? that the long-term consequences are unknown? The consequences of full versus limited disclosure became a theme in medical literature discussions (Zindrick 2000). Some disclosures seemed to distract from rather than help the patient focus on the most information about the procedure. Other information might serve to cause the patient to reject potentially beneficial surgery. How much information about the patient did a surgeon need to know before deciding how much to disclose? For instance, did surgeons need to know about patient assumptions—are they wary of new techniques or do they assume that all new procedures are better? Others wondered whether full disclosure would engender patient trust or undermine it. Is some information simply too sophisticated or difficult to convey accurately in the limited time a surgeon has with a patient? And—always a pertinent question—are some patients so desperate for a chance to survive that all disclosure becomes meaningless to the patient?

Case studies on patients who have accepted innovative surgery can make the situation real. Success stories are heartening, as when a patient is seen in a news story walking out of the hospital when, except for the courage of a pioneering surgeon, the person would have died.

> Israel Singer was slipping into a coma after suffering a stroke as his wife, Vicki, arrived at the hospital. "They took my daughter and me aside and suggested a D.N.R.—do not resuscitate," she recalled. "They said he would definitely die" or, at best, be in a vegetative state. But in a last-ditch effort, doctors at Columbia-Presbyterian Center in Manhattan lowered Mr. Singer's body temperature by blowing cold air over him and pumping frigid saltwater into his stomach. Mr. Singer, who lives in the Bronx, survived, and six years later, at 76, he reads British history and can walk a bit with a cane. Therapeutic hypothermia—reducing body temperature below normal—has faded in and out of fashion for 50 years, but it received a big endorsement last month when the American Heart Association published a recommendation that some victims of cardiac arrest be chilled. (Pollack 2003, p. 1)

Other stories are troubling and prompt one to ask what constitutes benefit and risk for patients who agree to have innovative surgery. James Quinn, a 52-year-old African American male with heart failure, was the fifth recipient of the AbioCor artificial heart, in late 2001. Quinn hoped the surgery would extend his life so that he could spend more time with his wife and grandchildren, but, except for a few short visits, he never again lived at home. Less than two months after the operation, Mr. Quinn had a stroke followed by a series of medical complications until a massive stroke caused his death, a little more than ten months after the initial surgery. The newspaper account of the story said in part,

> Mr. Quinn survived more than 60 days with his new heart, more than twice as long as he was expected to [have lived without it]. But his quality of life was poor. In an interview shortly before the stroke that killed him, Mr. Quinn, known as Butch, said that if he had to do it all over, he would stick with his natural heart. "This is nothing like I thought it would be," he said. "If I had to do it over again, I wouldn't do it. I would take my chances on life." . . . Dr. Samuels [the surgeon] wound up searching for "some solace, some reason to believe it was still worthwhile." . . . Mr. Berger

[the Abiomed company spokesman] said Abiomed was grateful to Mr. Quinn, who helped demonstrate the heart's reliability. . . . "You can say, 'Look what we achieved, it's positive,'" Mr. Berger said. "That is something you feel very good about. On the other hand, we want our patients to do well, and to feel that they are doing well." In that regard, he said, Mr. Quinn's story "is distressing." Dr. Samuels is not certain whether he will have another artificial heart patient. (Stolberg 2002, p. 1)

After Mr. Quinn's death, his widow sued the manufacturer of the device, the hospital where it was implanted, and a physician retained by the manufacturer who had served as Mr. Quinn's advocate. The lawsuit alleged that Mr. Quinn was not adequately informed of the consequences of consenting to the surgery.

Because of the impact on patients of innovative procedures, a third theme in the surgical literature was whether there should be more research on new procedures (Dossetor 1990; Brower 2003). As described earlier in this book, there are plenty of examples of accepted surgical procedures that have been abandoned when well-controlled research revealed either lack of efficacy or unacceptable risk. Yet, the surgeon's tendency is to introduce new procedures as innovative practice and not as research. The ethical ramifications of choosing this pathway include that patients may be harmed by subjecting themselves to procedures with unrevealed risks and that patients may not be told about the experimental nature of the procedures (Reitsma and Moreno 2002). Without an explicit and detailed experimental protocol, institutions and surgeons are apt to vary considerably in their selection of patients and choice of operative technique, as well as in their criteria for subsequent evaluation. As a result of this lack of consistency, it can take too long to determine the true value of new surgical techniques. Also, as one surgeon declared, once a case series using a new technique is presented at a scientific meeting or published, "there's no turning back" (Brower 2003); other surgeons will adopt it and continue to innovate on top of it.

Because of these concerns, commentators have long asked whether there should be FDA or some other kind of oversight and assessment process for surgical procedures (Spodick 1975; Bunker, Hinkley, and McDermott 1978). These suggestions inevitably elicit the arguments about the cumbersomeness, the delay, and the expense involved in IRB-controlled research. Modern academic physicians complain that it takes months to obtain an IRB review and months to obtain approval if changes are requested, and that the requirement to proceed under the strict confines of a research protocol introduces a rigidity that is unnatural and even harmful in the practice of surgery. When surgeons see a way to improve, they want to take it as soon as possible. Forcing comparisons in research slows innovation and, by the time the research is published, surgical processes have likely changed. It is also problematic to apply to surgery the gold standard randomized placebo-controlled study designs so valued in medicine, which would require placebo surgical procedures. Some commentators believe that the risks of placebo surgery are justified by the high rate of placebo response to surgical interventions. Others disagree, finding placebo-controlled surgery unacceptable because it does not minimize the risk of harm and has no benefit to the patient who is randomly assigned to the placebo arm of the study.

Surgical innovations often result from a nonlinear and unpredictable evolutionary cycle. This is why surgeons, more than most physicians, claim a need to retain flexibility to adapt to the ever-present anomalies that are encountered in the operating room. *King of Hearts* contains an example of the variability in the defects surgeons attempt to repair. In the process of developing a surgery for ventricular septal defects, Walton Lillehei, one of the early innovators of open-heart surgery, wanted to prepare himself for the types of lesion he would see in patients. At a Mayo Clinic pathology lab, Lillehei examined about fifty hearts with this particular defect and found no physical similarities that could inform him about the best surgical techniques to use. He concluded that the only way to approach ventricular septal surgery was to adapt his procedures to each patient, depending on what he found when he opened the heart.

At the time of this book's writing, surgeons are still trying to discover ways to perform coronary artery surgery without the problematic cardiopulmonary bypass machine (Heames et al. 2002). By 1999, new surgical tools (intracoronary shunts and special retractors) made this a possibility so long as the surgeon could learn how to operate on a beating heart. The possibility so excited two surgeons, Drs. Borst and Grundeman, that they predicted that, in five years, more than 50 percent of coronary surgery would be performed on the beating heart, mainly with arterial conduits, in part through limited access and, depending on costs, in part through the closed-chest approach. They recognized the great technical and surgical challenges involved in these procedures, but, for the sake of patient safety, urged the profession to continue to search for the solutions and develop the skills that would allow for this new surgical approach (Borst and Grundeman 1999). As surgeons continue this and other innovative processes, biomedical ethicists at the Center for Bioethics at the University of Virginia have begun a new initiative to attempt modern definitions of surgical innovation and recommend possible ways for it to be adopted by medical institutions (Reitsma 2003).

Dr. Wizbang is a cardiac surgeon with both medical and engineering degrees who devotes his academic career to improving the efficacy and safety of surgical procedures. He has made an international reputation as a surgical innovator. He holds many surgical device patents, and his surgical techniques and devices have routinely become standard in the cardiovascular field. His surgical program, which is based at a leading university teaching hospital, is regularly inundated with requests by other surgeons seeking training in advanced surgical techniques, and his residency program is one of the most popular in the country. Hospitals and surgeons know that if they can offer the advanced surgical procedures perfected by Dr. Wizbang, they can expand their practices and their professional revenues. Consequently, competition among these surgeons is intense.

Dr. Wizbang Innovates

Dr. W's newest innovation involves a technique and modified microsurgical devices for a new form of noninvasive cardiac surgery. This system is intended to allow surgeons to perform heart surgery without opening the chest or stopping the heart. Many of the complications and most of the trauma, pain, and rehabilitation time of cardiac surgery are attributed to the need to cut open the chest from the clavicle to the abdomen, aplit apart the breastbone, and spread open the ribcage to expose the heart. To eliminate the open-chest complications, Dr. W and other surgeons had previously developed surgical devices and techniques that allowed many of the same surgeries to be performed with closed-chest or minimally invasive techniques, using mini-cameras and surgical tools on wires that are passed to the heart through several small incisions in the chest wall.

Dr. W's current innovation allows him to avoid both the open-chest and the bypass complications. He has perfected in animals the ability to perform closed-chest cardiac surgeries while the heart is still beating. This is considered a major achievement but takes considerable surgical skill, because operating on a beating heart makes it much more difficult to cut, guide instruments, and sew with precision. Dr. W's breakthroughs are especially important because cardiac surgeries are more often performed on older and sicker patients, who are at higher risk from both the open-chest and the bypass procedures. Dr. W is looking forward to introducing his new techniques and to the resultant decline in mortality and morbidity associated with many cardiovascular surgical procedures.

1. Should the first people who submit to surgical procedures be considered research subjects or patients?
2. Does Dr. W have a responsibility to submit his surgical procedure innovations to the medical school IRB and proceed with his initial human surgeries under a research protocol? What would be gained by going this route? What lost?
3. Even if he does not proceed under an IRB-approved research protocol, does Dr. W have an obligation (to the surgical profession? to prospective patients?) to collect and disseminate clinical practice outcome data on his new procedure?

The Surgical Devices

The surgical tools developed by Dr. W for the new procedure are submitted for FDA approval through a process in which the devices are shown to be substantially equivalent to approved marketed devices used for closed-chest surgery. This FDA approval process does not require that the devices undergo safety and efficacy testing in humans before implementation. The devices are eligible for this accelerated approval process because Dr. W modified existing approved devices to fit the needs of beating-heart surgery. The device innovations, used in varying numbers and ways, are coupled with Dr. W's advances in surgical technique, which are not dependent upon a formal regulation process.

The device approval application is being sponsored by a company formed by Dr. W. He raised venture capital funds to create the company and sell the new devices in a surgical set, the first of which will be marketed for use in coronary artery bypass graft surgeries. (The market for these surgeries is growing as the population grows older. By age 60, one of every three men and one of every ten women show clinical signs of coronary artery disease and are potential candidates for CABG procedures.) So many of these procedures were being done that the company consultants believe that yearly sales of the surgical kits could exceed $750 million.

As a company founder, Dr. W was issued stock options, he took a seat on the board, and he continues to advise the company. However, he is not active in day-to-day operations, preferring to spend his time in academic medicine. Because of Dr. W's other commitments, he is unable to spend as much time with the company as planned and it takes longer than expected for the company to perfect the quality control necessary to manufacture Dr. W's devices. Eventually, some small modifications cure the quality control problems and the devices are approved for sale by the FDA. However, Dr. W keeps rejecting the devices produced by the company, preferring to use his own. Although company managers assert that there is no significant difference between company tools and those from his lab, Dr. W maintains that only he knows the import of the discrepancies. This frustrates company managers, who need to get products to market, given that cash reserves are dwindling and the board of directors is reluctant to dilute share ownership by seeking a second round of financing. The company managers seek the advice of other surgeons, some of whom trained with Dr. W, and are told that the company's devices are perfectly acceptable for the intended purpose. Some of the feedback also suggests that Dr. W's recalcitrance is due not to quality problems but to general business disagreements with his corporate partners. One such disagreement involves the company's plan to assemble a surgical training team for new surgeon customers, and some suspect that Dr. W's ego has convinced him that no one can train others to do the procedure as well as he can.

4. What does this case suggest about the impact of academic-corporate collaborations on the introduction of novel medical technologies?

Surgical Success and Training

Dr. W begins to operate on cardiac patients using his new procedure, and his results become the marvel of the cardiovascular surgical field. His CABG success rates, at first lower than the national norm, have risen to well above normal. Similarly, his rates of adverse surgical events, although initially higher, have fallen to well below the norm. In the past several hundred patients, no deaths have been attributed to the procedures he performed, whereas national statistics suggest that there could have been as many as four deaths attributable to surgical procedures. Hospital time and postoperative rehabilitation are significantly shorter than for Dr. W's prior CABG patients. Patients are now coming from everywhere for the procedure and the wait list is growing. This situation pleases the hospital administrators immensely, and they begin to market the fact that theirs is the only hospital in the world where this procedure is performed. In addition to the safety and efficacy benefits, the hospital touts the fact that the hospital bill is often much lower than with the conventional surgical technique; despite the fact that physician fees are higher, the overall cost of the procedure is up to $10,000 less than CABG at other hospitals. Those of Dr. W's surgical residents who have completed their training then start to perform the new CABG procedure at other hospitals, further increasing the popularity of the surgery.

In the meantime, the manufacturing company knows that Dr. W is making an important point when he claims that he alone has the skills to obtain the results he is getting and to train others. If the devices are to be a success, other surgeons will need to develop a comparable level of skill. Research has consistently shown that higher CABG surgical volume correlates to better clinical outcomes and lower death rates, for both hospitals and surgeons. Therefore, surgeon customers of the company will need to be trained to a certain level of skill and achieve a certain amount of experience so that the company can successfully sell its surgical tool kits. One of the important aspects of the training is making surgeons comfortable with the surgical microscope cameras developed for the procedure. Along with ultrasound equipment, several of these are needed for surgeons to visualize the area of operation. These cameras are connected to monitors suspended above the operating table, requiring the surgeons continually to look up at the monitor while manipulating the instruments inside the patient's chest. Dr. W has become very adept at this visually and tactilely indirect process, as have most of the new generation of surgical residents. However, the majority of veteran cardiac surgeons are familiar with direct visualization techniques, the ones used in open-chest procedures. Those who have some familiarity with arthroscopic surgical procedures do not have training in the use of the multiple cameras, and they need to acquire quick reflexes to operate on a beating heart. The company knows that the market for the surgical took kits, therefore, depends on the number of surgeons who can adapt to the new tools and techniques before they start performing human surgeries. One other complication that the company faces is that, as Dr. W keeps doing these surgeries, he is continually modifying and improving his own methods and tweaking his tools accordingly. And he has very little time to update the corporate training team.

5. Given the need for skill development, what should the company do to ensure that its products are used safely and effectively? Should the company be the sole determiner of how the new tools and techniques are introduced into medical practice? What responsibilities do physicians and hospitals have in this process? Are there other entities or organizations that should participate? Should there be any formal, enforceable procedures?

Selection of Patients

There is a growing demand for Dr. W's new procedure. Among these prospective patients there is much variety in age, health, and susceptibility to complications from the surgery. Many of the surgeons trained to use the devices for this new surgery are eager to set up their own programs to provide beating-heart, closed-chest procedures.

6. What kind of patients should be selected for the first cases in these new programs?
7. What should the physician disclose to patients with regard to his or her experience with the new procedure? For instance, should surgeons disclose that they are on a learning curve or that other surgeons may have more experience and therefore better outcomes? As a matter of policy, should patients bear the burden of asking about these issues, or should surgeons volunteer such information?
8. Whose responsibility is it to determine what disclosures are appropriate?

Surgeons' Experience and Company Response

News of the innovative procedure and its potential benefits spreads after Dr. W publishes his post–learning curve results. The company is busily putting surgeon customers through a costly training program (using live pigs as surgical models) and assisting with and monitoring the outcomes of the first surgeries on humans. In the beginning, more surgeons applied for the training than could be accommodated, despite the fact that the company had been able to introduce efficiencies and streamline its training program from four and a half days to two and a half days. After one year's experience, company executives have good news and bad news. The marketing campaign was initially very successful, and physician and hospital demand for the training and surgical tool kit was higher than expected. Some of the surgeons have embraced the new technique and are reporting outcomes that approach those of Dr. W. The hospitals where these surgeons practice have become magnets for patients seeking the improved outcomes. However, other surgeons have begun to complain that the procedure takes much longer than expected, placing patients at greater anesthesia risk; outcomes are sometimes worse than for the conventional surgery; and there have been some surgical injuries. Those surgeons with disappointing results have either given up and returned to open-chest procedures or continue to complain to the company that it has not done enough to prepare surgeon trainees, especially because they keep hearing of Dr. W's modified techniques, which they feel have been withheld from company training.

When company executives question their unhappy customers about the objections, most comments relate to a few themes: that dissatisfactions are caused by learning curve issues, that the surgeons lack good supporting OR teams, that professional jealousy exists regarding colleagues with better outcomes, and that some surgeons are blaming the company for inadequate training. In addition, some surgeons and hospitals complain that the company charges too much for the training, holding them hostage, since they are not able otherwise to obtain the training. Clearly, it is not feasible for the company to extensively retrain its surgeon customers or to tailor training to individuals with different OR setups. But, where is the line between enough training and too little? The company is troubled by the lack of uniformity in both physician acceptance and outcomes and by the fact that sales, initially high, have recently started to fall below projected levels. Company investors are becoming restless about the drop in company performance and the overall failure of the company to return a profit. In addition, the company board is nervous that, if even one of the injured patients sues, the legal damages could result in a severe financial setback for this fledgling company.

9. Because the devices cannot be marketed without training in the associated surgical techniques, what does this case suggest about the role of corporations in the introduction into medical practice of innovative surgical devices and techniques?

10. Whose responsibility is it to protect the interests of patients potentially imperiled by the introduction of new surgical techniques that aim to replace well-established procedures?

CHAPTER FIVE

Innovation in Assisted Reproduction

THE BACKGROUND

Assisted reproductive technology (ART) had its start in the 1970s and, according to estimates by the Centers for Disease Control and Prevention (CDC), since 1978 approximately 0.9 percent of all U.S. births and more than one million children worldwide have been conceived with ART procedures. Until the late 1980s, assisted reproductive technology was successful only 10 percent of the time. However, by 2000, success rates were slightly more than 35 percent for the 383 U.S. clinics reporting data to the CDC (99,639 ART cycles resulted in 35,025 live babies born). The perceived safety and success of assisted reproductive technology has led to an increasing demand for its use. Responding to the demand, the number of fertility specialists and clinics has grown, increasing the competition for patients. This competition has led to assertive marketing of fertility services to referring doctors and directly to consumers, as well as to reductions in cost, with some clinics offering financing programs and money-back guarantees. In the United States, the infertility treatment industry grosses $2 billion per year, with couples paying up to $200,000 to achieve a single pregnancy (Andrews 1999; Kolata 2002; Centers for Disease Control and Prevention 2003).

The field of assisted reproductive technology is noted for its constant innovations. It started with in vitro fertilization, or IVF, treatment.[1] Over time, IVF has been modified with techniques such as gamete intrafallopian transfer (GIFT),[2] zygote intrafallopian transfer (ZIFT),[3] and intracytoplasmic sperm injection (ICSI).[4]

Because 50 to 80 percent of embryos produced via IVF have been chromosomally abnormal, preimplantation genetic diagnosis was recently introduced, and this development has also significantly advanced the field. In preimplantation genetic diagnosis, a technician removes a cell or two from the developing embryos and tests for the sex of the embryo and for genetic abnormalities, so that only embryos free of certain sex-linked or genetic defects are used to impregnate the mother.

To accomplish these ART procedures, highly sophisticated and microminiaturized tools and special culture media and freezing techniques have been developed; highly skilled technicians are required to perform the work. Frequently the new tools are made in the lab of the innovator. Also, the procedural innovations are introduced as practice modifications rather than as controlled research, in part because U.S. laws forbid any federal agency to fund research involving human embryos. The political climate surrounding assisted reproductive technology has left it without federal regulation in the United States except for mandatory reporting of pregnancy success rates, which has been criticized as unverified, inconsistent, and unreliable. Neither are there comprehensive or specific state regulations. Instead, the field is guided by voluntary and unenforced professional standards published by two professional societies, the American Society of Reproductive Medicine and the American College of Obstetricians and Gynecologists. These guidelines specify minimum standards for IVF and some other related procedures, and these standards have been cited in some but not all medicolegal settings as the standard of care.

Many of the physicians (it is difficult to learn how many) who practice IVF are board certified in reproductive endocrinology and infertility. The ART labs are also usually (again, the number is uncertain) certified under general laboratory procedure standards and, depending on the circumstances and the jurisdiction, under tissue bank regulations. There is, as well, the voluntary Reproductive Laboratory Accreditation Program, which has developed guidelines for lab personnel qualifications, resource and facility requirements, quality control and assurance, record keeping, and proficiency testing. In addition, most IVF practitioners participate in the Society for Assisted Reproductive Technologies, which maintains a registry on the outcomes of ART procedures and periodically analyzes the registry data to develop further practice recommendations.

Whether assisted reproductive technology should be regulated any further is the subject of ongoing debate. Proponents see the need to curb irresponsible use of unproven techniques and to ensure proper consent. Opponents, including some infertility advocacy groups, fear that legislation and regulation will interfere with medical practice and patients' rights, increase the cost of treatment, limit access to treatment, and politicize medical and personal choices (Adamson 2002; Marcus 2002).

Given the nature of in vitro fertilization (treatment cycles take more than a month, a pregnancy takes nine months, and the children produced take years to mature), understanding whether treatment modifications have succeeded, failed, or produced problems can take a long time. The fact that serious complications are rare and can be subtle makes this assessment even more difficult. Nonetheless, the scientists and physicians who advance the field are always concerned that innovations not injure the egg and sperm, the mother, or the resulting baby and child (Korean 2002).

Problems high on the list of concern for physicians in the field include that the culture medium in which the embryo is formed and grows not produce abnormalities. Instruments used in ART are also constantly revised to reduce the incidence of damage to gametes and embryos. The incidence of multiple births from IVF is also problematic. In most cases, to increase the chance of one successful birth, more than one embryo is implanted in the woman's uterus. However, this increases the risk of multiple births. Carrying multiple fetuses increases the risks of pregnancy and the risk that a child or the children will be born under weight (less that 2,500 g). Underweight infants are prone to a host of medical problems, and some die. It is uncertain whether IVF also increases the risk of low birth weight among single-birth infants.

Birth defects related to ART are of special concern. A major question has been whether birth defects could be a result of the procedure itself, be associated with the multiple births that commonly result from IVF, or be related to the often older age of women who use ART. In 1996, after data had been collected and analyzed, the American Society of Reproductive Medicine felt confident in reporting that IVF did not increase the risk of birth defects (American Society of Reproductive Medicine 1996). However, other physicians worried that existing studies were insufficiently precise, that birth defects in IVF infants were either underreported or overreported. In addition, some studies showing no increased incidence were suspected of lacking a similarly screened comparison group. Neither did U.S. data seem to jibe with data from other countries. One later Australian study in particular was worrisome, for it showed that, by one year of age, one or more major birth defects had been identified in 9.0 percent of babies conceived with ART, compared with 4.2 percent of those who were conceived naturally (Mitchell 2002). Inconsistent findings such as these trouble physicians, because it is always difficult to determine whose data are more accurate and why discrepancies exist (Lambert 2002).

Preimplantation genetic diagnosis has also challenged the field of assisted reproductive technology. No one doubts the benefits of being able to prevent the implantation of genetically defective embryos. One account of the use of preimplantation genetic diagnosis is enough to convince. The *Wall Street Journal* carried a story about a woman, Jennifer Francis, who had a genetic defect that carried with it a 90 percent chance of miscarriage. She had been trying to conceive for two years. Doctors in her case used preimplantation genetic diagnosis to look for genetic defects or missing critical chromosomes in her embryos. "In the Francises' case, all of the embryos produced had too few or too many chromosomes—except for one. 'That's our baby, Ruby,' now six months old, Mrs. Francis says. 'I've got the baby in my arms, and you can't put a price tag on that'" (Johannes 2004, p. D1).

However, disputes have risen over the safety of preimplantation genetic diagnosis (Does it damage the embryo? Will newer, less experienced labs derive accurate results?) and over the extent of use (Is it overused? Should it be used to identify the gender of the child or to select for certain genetic traits that enhance life rather than eliminate a disease? Should it be used to create babies to be compatible cell donors for sick siblings?). So far, about 1,500 babies have been born using preimplantation genetic diagnosis, and the reliability has improved to the point where physicians believe that nine out of ten embryos with defects can be detected. These statistics and the utility of preimplantation genetic diagnosis are sure to improve as test innovation continues.

Not only must potential parents seeking IVF contend with adverse effect uncertainties, they must also decide whether they can endure the procedures. Assisted reproductive technology is a daunting process, requiring immense dedication on the part of all participants—those people seeking to produce a baby and the professionals helping them. Often months of treatment and many failures precede a successful pregnancy. In 2002, Michael Ryan wrote an account of his and his wife's experience of conceiving and giving birth to a child using assisted reproduction after a "Rubik's cube of permutations" had failed to produce a pregnancy. Ryan began his account this way:

> I have been telling my friends that what I am injecting into my wife, Doreen, this week is crushed, powdered Chinese hamster ovaries. This is not quite the truth. I am injecting her with cells from Chinese hamster ovaries that have been genetically

reengineered to help develop multiple eggs and, in thirty-three per cent of the live births that result, multiple babies: twins, triplets, quadruplets, and up. It's called Gonal-F, and it costs $3,674.50 for a full course of treatment—one injection a day for twelve days during the first half of the menstrual cycle. This is just one element of the in-vitro treatment that Doreen and I hope will give us a baby.

Ryan goes on to describe a harrowing experience of repeated failed attempts to achieve pregnancy that ultimately results in his wife's becoming pregnant with triplet embryos, a very high risk condition. Subsequently, one of the triplets divides to produce a fourth, at which point "reductions" are required to eliminate what are believed to be the low-probability embryos. Ryan ends his account, however, on a very happy note: "We are the lucky people. Emily elicits a tenderness in me I hadn't known before she was born, not to mention an anxiety for her well-being that makes my other fears seem about as threatening as cocker spaniel puppies. And the joy of watching Doreen with her is beyond what I could have imagined; I never had tried to imagine it, because the risk of not experiencing it would have been too much" (Ryan 2002).

Ryan's account is not unlike that of others who have struggled through the process and ended up with a living, healthy baby. The story is typical of couples who seek IVF as a last resort to a desperately sought biological parenthood. It is interesting that Ryan's account does not contain much in the way of acknowledgment of the dangers of IVF procedures. This could be because the account was written after a successful outcome in which everyone was healthy. It could also be that people who consent to ART do not want to acknowledge the risks. Physicians engaged in ART confirm that many patients focus much more on the success rates than on the risks and other negative information presented to them in the consent process. Ryan's story also makes it easy to see that both success and failure with IVF can produce intense emotions. According to Pamela Madison, executive director of the American Infertility Association, a national support organization, couples are often full of hope at the beginning. If, after several treatment cycles, there is no pregnancy, hope begins to fade and, commonly, the fear of failure sets in. Repeated failure to conceive or the loss of an established pregnancy can too often cause chronic grief and depression (Tarkan 2002).

Given the widespread expansion of ART services, the frequency of innovative change in the field, and the consequences to patients, some commentators have become uneasy about the rapidity and ease with which ART techniques have been transformed from experimental to therapeutic status. The whole process is driven by the strong need to procreate, and those who can afford the service often search for and demand the newer techniques (Blank 1997). The pace and demand suggest to some that more caution is warranted so that advances are not adopted without full understanding of the safety and social implications, especially for the children. Proposed solutions have included governmental regulations; multidisciplinary commissions of lay people and professionals to study the need for regulation and to make recommendations; physician, technician, and lab accreditation; and/or comprehensive legislation (Lorio 1999; Charo 2002; Johnson 2002; Petersen 2002). Objections to all of these consumer-protection proposals have also been posed. The government, some say, should not intervene in such a private area of human behavior, where reproductive liberty rights exist. Further, the medical profession and the policies for the reimbursement of health services are sufficient to prevent harm, especially because insurance coverage of therapies is often predicated on proof of efficacy and safety. The malpractice system is another deterrent to reckless practices. Besides, objectors say, regulations are not needed; the field has progressed safely so far and the anticipated harms are only speculative in nature. Others object to the delay caused by any comprehensive review. Commission work and consensus building is a slow process, and by the time any commission makes recommendations, the underlying science and technology have usually moved on. Objections exist to accreditation or a licensing process that requires specific training and demonstration of quality, because such an approach to protecting patient safety offers no practice guidelines. Legislation is also problematic. Comprehensive legislation often fosters more restrictive and intrusive regulation and often lags behind technological progress. Others say that any legislative debate on the regulation of assisted reproductive technology will be hijacked by and subsumed in the abortion debate and, hence, will go nowhere. Objectors to any form of external control favor a market-driven or peer-regulated approach that, most importantly, needs to operate without hindering the progress that has so far resulted in the birth of more than one million children to infertile couples. At the time that the case below was written, no consensus had risen from this mix of views about whether there should be greater oversight of ART, and the debates remain active.

THE CASE STUDY

The Genesis Fertility Clinic is a privately owned facility offering assisted reproductive services. These include artificial insemination and surrogacy services, but the issues presented by this case involve in vitro fertilization technology, including egg harvesting, embryo culture, preimplantation diagnosis, and cryogenic embryo preservation. Genesis is led by Dr. Oldwest, a confident, experienced physician with a reputation for clinical innovation and an aggressive concern for his patients. Mr. and Mrs. Hopeful (the H's) arrive at Genesis after a history of unsuccessful efforts to conceive and accompanied by medical histories confirming that Mr. H's sperm are viable. While the cause of their infertility has never been specifically determined, the couple is desperate to conceive and bear a child of their own, and they request IVF. Dr. O explains that it should be possible to achieve IVF by inducing multiple ovulation through hormone injections and aspirating the ova, which would then be fertilized with Mr. H's sperm in a special culture medium. Some of the embryos would then be introduced into Mrs. H's uterus while others would be cryogenically preserved.

The Doctor

Genesis has its own assisted reproduction lab where the embryos are developed and cultured before transfer into the uterus of the female patient or surrogate. Dr. O and his colleagues have known since the beginning of this venture that the media employed to culture embryos in vitro are extremely important to the pregnancy success rates achievable with the embryos. The culture formulations are responsible for adequately nurturing the new embryo and promoting rapid and healthy development so that sufficient embryos are produced that have a maximal chance of creating a pregnancy. Dr. O avidly follows the scientific literature and is eager to apply advances in embryo culture; thus, over time, the culture media used in Dr. O's lab have become complex and are always state-of-the-art. Dr. O has been careful, however, to make only those changes in the lab's culture media that, in his opinion, have been shown to be effective and safe in studies on laboratory mammals and that are consistent with what is known about the human pregnant state. Recently, his colleagues have incorporated into the lab's formulas some growth factors that have been shown in multiple animal studies to support embryo growth in culture for longer periods of time. This produces more mature and thus more viable embryos, promising higher pregnancy rates with fewer embryos, making pregnancy safer for both mother and fetus. Dr. O is so confident of the superiority of these new culture media that he has filed for patent protection for the formulas and believes that he may be able to generate substantial licensing revenue from the sale of his formulations via a separate commercial venture. He has also submitted manuscripts to a prestigious medical journal to inform the medical community of his innovations.

One problem has appeared in responses written to the scientific publications by some embryologists saying that growth factors of the class used by Dr. O might cause abnormalities in children born of an IVF procedure using these culture ingredients. However, Dr. O considers these fears to be highly speculative; such fears are expressed whenever new ingredients are added to embryo culture media, and they have become almost an obligatory caution added to the end of scientific papers disclosing animal advances in this field. The growth factors used by Dr. O are those that are produced by the newly pregnant human female and are, therefore, ones to which the embryo would be exposed under normal conditions. Thus, Dr. O believes that he is creating a more physiologically normal environment for the embryos created in his lab. Over the past year, Dr. O has used the culture media in his last eleven IVF procedures, and all four infants born from those procedures have been healthy and normal.

1. Should Dr. O's culture work be considered research or clinical practice? Is it ethical for Dr. O to "test" his own invention on his own patients? If so, under what conditions?

2. Should work such as Dr. O's be subject to regulatory oversight? How, and by what body or bodies?

3. Dr. O has been invited to present a paper at a symposium on assisted reproductive technology. He intends to report his experience with his new culture media. What are his disclosure responsibilities in this paper?

4. Is Dr. O obliged to report his past use of and his experience with his modified culture media and the speculative risks to the Hopeful family as part of an informed consent procedure? What, specifically, should he disclose?

5. Is Dr. O obliged to disclose his financial interest in the culture media he is using? What about his reputational interests?

The Patients

Dr. O shows Mr. and Mrs. H an informed consent form. It explains the risks of the hormonal treatments used to induce ovulation and those associated with the aspiration of the ova. It also supplies information about "failure rates" of the IVF procedure as a whole. Mrs. H has read extensively about the procedure on the Internet, and she asks about the risks associated with multiple births; Dr. O explains that, to increase the success rate for the procedure, he must implant multiple embryos. Multiple births pose some risk to the mother and increase the likelihood that one or more of the siblings may have low birth weight. Dr. O then summarizes the risks associated with low birth weight, but points out that pregnancy termination would be an option if that were a prospect. Mrs. H discloses that she would have a very difficult time agreeing to the termination of the life of any living implanted embryo. Dr. O goes on to explain that because her genetic history suggests certain risks, her embryos should be subjected to preimplantation genetic diagnosis so that those carrying identifiable defects could be eliminated. Even though preimplantation genetic diagnosis is very expensive (sometimes equaling the cost of the IVF procedure), he tells the couple that he would be reluctant to perform IVF without doing the testing because the ability to diagnose problems in embryos will greatly increase the chance of producing a healthy child. Genesis routinely does these tests on embryos, storing the sampled tissue for future reference. Dr. O states that, although he will explain these tests to them, given the complexity of the matter, the decisions of what tests are reliable enough to employ and which embryos to select for implantation should be left to his discretion.

Dr. O has just encountered some data that, if true, would probably apply to the Hopefuls. He read a recently published report of a medical study conducted by British researchers that showed that normal-weight children born of IVF techniques have a higher incidence of neurological abnormalities than those born naturally. However, the study's conclusions had been criticized because of the relatively low number of children studied and the fact that the study failed to resolve the question of whether the increase in abnormalities was caused by the infertility procedures or the infertility itself or some other factors. Furthermore, it was difficult to extrapolate British results to the United States because some of the techniques used in IVF in the two countries differ. Based on these uncertainties, Dr. O has decided not to disclose this confusing information to his patients.

6. Should the consent form and/or Dr. O's explanation also include the epidemiological uncertainty associated with later life in those IVF children who are normal with respect to birth weight?

7. What evidence should be in place to require such a duty to disclose? Would the British study qualify in this instance?

8. How much control over the IVF process is Dr. O justified in maintaining, and to what extent should the patients participate in such medical decisions as what preimplantation genetic diagnosis tests to employ, which embryos, and how many, should be selected for implantation? Whose interests are at stake in these decisions?

The Parents, Later

Mr. and Mrs. Hopeful indicate that they would like the medical record to state that their consent to IVF is conditioned on Dr. O's agreement and that of the clinic's administration to the following conditions: that any viable, healthy embryos that are not implanted will be cryogenically preserved; that Mr. and Mrs. H will be jointly responsible for decisions about the future use and custody of their frozen embryos; and that no genetic information obtained through preimplantation genetic diagnosis or any other means will be shared with another person or entity (including but not limited to an insurance carrier). With some reluctance about the third condition, Dr. O agrees. The IVF is successful. Multiple embryos develop and look reasonably viable. Some are cryopreserved and three embryos are implanted. Three pregnancies result, two of which are eliminated in utero because Dr. O determined that Mrs. H's subsequently developed pregnancy problems put her at high risk with a multiple gestation. The decision to undergo the pregnancy-reduction procedure was very difficult for Mrs. H. She had consulted with her religious advisor, her husband, and her sisters. After much anguished contemplation, she agreed to termination based on Dr. O's assurance that the risks of multiple pregnancies were medically unacceptable for her and for the one fetus selected for retention. Although Mrs. H recognizes that Dr. O had discussed with her in advance the risks of multiple pregnancies, she cannot help repeating her wish that she had fully understood, from the beginning, the impact of making the reduction decision. She also says that her joy connected with the anticipation of birth is significantly diminished because of her distress over the thought of those two "lost babies."

9. When research conducted subsequent to this procedure implicates a particular genetic marker in an important medical disorder, Dr. O runs the new genetic test on all of the preserved embryo tissue in his lab (he has stored more than one thousand samples) and finds the marker in Baby H's tissue. Because of the importance to medical understanding and the public health, Dr. O wants to release the data for incorporation into a national database along with medical information about the Hopefuls. How should he proceed?

10. Dr. O also wonders what his obligations are concerning informing the H's about this finding in Baby H's tissue. Does this suggest that Dr. O should have considered his testing of the stored tissues as research and

obtained prior consent from the H's? Aside from any new privacy obligations under HIPAA,[5] what would constitute prudent practice when physicians obtain, store, and then test human tissue, as in this case?

11. If Dr. O does inform the H's about the genetic finding, they will learn that
there is an association between the presence of the genetic marker and the
development of a particular type of mental disorder. In addition to informing the H's about potential health risks, does Dr. O have a duty to mitigate the harms (including psychological and social) that the H's might
experience as a result of learning about the genetic test findings?

The Child, Much Later

Baby Hopeful, named Ernest, is now 19. Over his lifetime, there have been
subtle indications that he was not normal neurologically. His doctors have tested
him periodically and noted mild cognitive deficits, but, because his verbal, social, emotional, and other scores improved as he aged, doctors advised the Hopefuls that their child would score within the normal range by the end of adoles-
cence. However, the cognitive test scores never quite reached a normal range and
have remained set since the age of 15. Ernest's condition now has a name, high-
functioning autism syndrome, or HFAS; it is considered a form of childhood
developmental disability, a variant of autism that had previously fallen into a category of unclassified disorders called Pervasive Developmental Disorder–Not
Otherwise Specified (PDD–NOS). HFAS has left Ernest somewhat socially withdrawn with weak communication skills and some emotional lability. These problems presage difficulties with education, employment, and social interactions.
On the advice of legal counsel, Ernest has sued his physicians for failing to diagnose this condition in a timely manner. Among the list of injuries claimed is a
lost opportunity to engage in therapy when it had the best chance of success. His
lawyers know that this is a potentially viable claim only because researchers have
not yet identified a single "trigger" for autism but among the nongenetic possibilities are early embryonic or fetal exposure to chemicals and other nonphysio-
logical substances. To increase the chances of prevailing in their claim, Ernest's
lawyers are also suing Dr. O and the Genesis Clinic, on the theory that the IVF
procedure carried risks that were, or should have been, known by Dr. O but were
not properly disclosed to the H's in the informed consent process. Dr. O has substantially changed the embryo culture formulations that were used in the IVF
that produced Ernest. Because it was likely that the claim against Dr. O would be

dismissed as a legally disfavored "wrongful life" claim, a second legal theory against Dr. O was newly developed for this lawsuit. According to the pleading, Dr. O should be punished for failing to treat his patients as research subjects, which was akin to acting in reckless disregard for Ernest's health and well-being by performing the IVF itself and/or by using untested culture media. If the culture formulations had been treated as experimental, the lawsuit papers claim, there would have been more extensive preclinical testing and more human subject protections in place that would have protected Ernest from premature exposure to the damaging embryo culture chemicals.

12. Increasingly, courts are asked to address claims relating to evolving medical understanding. In addition, medical advances or the implementation of new medical technologies can lead to novel alleged harms, in turn generating new legal theories to redress them. What can society do to prepare courts for such novel cases?

13. How could such potential after-the-fact tangles be avoided prospectively by the clinic and the parents? What features of the process would require structural change?

CHAPTER SIX

Innovation in Neuroimaging

THE BACKGROUND

Functional magnetic resonance imaging (fMRI) is a new medical tool that is being used to understand diseases of the brain and nervous system and also the neural basis for human behavior. Findings from fMRI and other neuroimaging techniques produce real-time images that show which parts of the brain are active at that time. For instance, fMRI images can detect when parts of the brain controlling memory are activated.[1] Using these new imaging techniques, investigators can study brain function in people with conditions such as dementia or with maladaptive behaviors such as drug abuse. The knowledge gained through these images can suggest new avenues for treatment. Eventually, neuroimaging will be used to generate information about how the brain works in such situations as responding to drugs, learning new skills, remembering facts, recognizing faces, experiencing pain, telling lies, and responding to gestures of love, hostility, or trauma. While MRI machines require approval under FDA device regulations, the use to which they are put is largely governed by professional practice standards, and physicians are free to deploy new uses as medical practice or under a research protocol.

Of the technologies described in this book, fMRI is the newest, so people are less able to predict the consequences of its use. In addition, there are concerns about the technology's impact on the essence of the human condition, as there were early on with genetics. Stanford University law professor Hank Greely (2002) raised a question about functional neuroimaging that sets the stage for the discussion that follows: "Essentialism is a more interesting issue in neuroscience than in genetics. . . . I am more than my genes. The genes are an important part of me, but I can be certain that they are not my essence; they are not my soul. When we shift that notion to the neuroscience area, though, I am not so confident. Is my consciousness—is my brain—me? I am tempted to think it is" (p. 88). If Greely is right about how personal and fundamental neuroimaging information is, the consequences of its use need careful attention. Also, neuroimaging is rapidly evolving, making it likely that questions about deployment as research or clinical practice will attach to this technology as with the others described in this book.

The first specific questions being asked about the use of fMRI include whether images are reliable and whether they can be responsibly applied in medicine. In the early 2000s, researchers are just beginning to make correlations between images, mental activity, and behavior, and what to make of these correlations will continue to be challenging for a long time. For instance, given that the spectrum of human behavior is broad, defining what is normal and abnormal brain activity will have to be determined very carefully (Illes et al. 2003). What if someone with no symptoms is found by neuroimaging to have a tendency toward aberrant mental activity? And statistical differences in brain images will have to be correlated, not just with definitions of disease, but also with cultural and value-laden determinations of normality. These will come into play when studying such things as moral reasoning, deception, and sexual responsiveness.

The next big topic being addressed involves the use of brain-imaging information. How much screening should be allowed? Should brain imaging remain a medical technology, or does it have other legitimate uses? Eventually, most technology experts expect that the existence of fMRI data will invite the possibility of altering neurological traits to control illness, alter personality, or improve brain function. This possibility raises safety and social and ethical concerns.

Access to and protection of fMRI data is a third big issue. Medical information is subject to a number of state and federal privacy protections, and it is tempting to assume that neuroimaging information falls under the same privacy protections. But, what if the imaging is not done to diagnose or treat a disease? And, given the sensitivity of the information revealed, are the existing privacy laws adequate? People already refuse to be tested for genetic predisposition to disease because they do not want to lose their employment or insurance or they don't want to ruin their chances for marriage. Neuroimaging information could be just as socially damaging.

Professionals who venture into the territory of neuroimaging will have an impact on how and when the technology will be deployed and on how the issues of legitimate use and privacy will be addressed. Because neuroimaging reveals how the brain works in diseased and healthy patients, psychiatrists and psychologists will be heavy users of the technology, as both researchers and clinicians. Social scientists will obviously also want to use fMRI to study human behavior. Neurosurgeons will want the images in order to determine what areas to target or avoid when performing brain surgery to repair, destroy, or transplant brain tissue. Lawyers and judges will most likely become interested in the technology when, as many predict, fMRI data are submitted as evidence of criminal culpability or innocence. And there may be others who want to know how we think so that they can take commercial advantage of the information.

Considering only the uses described above, one can see that a host of medical, ethical, legal, and social issues will attach to fMRI applications. Will the data be used to define normalcy or personal identity? Can the data be used for social control? Will the data tend to stigmatize people? Questions such as these make it clear to many professional users of the technology that there is a need to identify specific standards for brain research and neuroscience and their clinical applications (Gindro and Mordini 1998).

At the time the case below was written, commentators were already addressing these issues and offering suggestions on what standards should apply to the use of neuroimaging technology. A bioethicist from the University of Virginia, Dr. Jonathan Moreno, presented an example of a dilemma that made it difficult to know if the physician should hold off on using the technology in certain cases (Moreno 2003). He posits the following: neuroimaging can detect a lesion associated with Alzheimer disease years before a patient has symptoms and before the discovery of effective therapies for the disease.

A number of those at risk for Alzheimer disease might request brain imaging. Some clinicians will view testing for risk status as appropriate, arguing that it will facilitate long-term planning, whereas others will urge that any such detection should only take place as part of a clinical trial until a medical intervention is available. Some consensus will be required concerning appropriate counseling in such cases. In these circumstances, we can learn from history. When presymptomatic diagnosis for Huntington disease became available, some expected a rush to testing. But in the absence of an adequate intervention, many have opted against knowing their genetically determined destiny. If ignorance is not exactly bliss, neither is knowledge in the absence of a solution. (p. 152)

Other commentators (Canli and Amin 2002) discussed the consequences of fMRI's being used to develop new approaches to the prevention or treatment of social ills. For instance, researchers have compared functional brain activity in normal, healthy individuals (affective neuroimaging) with imaging from violent, psychopathic individuals (forensic neuroimaging). To no one's surprise, there were differences. Another study, at Yale University in 2000, looked at whether brain imaging could detect unconscious racism in white students. Students who reported no conscious racism were scanned, and the images showed that the amygdala, which generates and registers fear and is associated with emotional learning, was more active when students were shown unfamiliar black faces than unfamiliar white faces. The same students showed no amygdala response to familiar black faces. Some have interpreted the data from such studies as showing a biological basis for socially relevant issues, in these cases, violent behavior and racism. However, the commentators caution against a naïve acceptance of the conclusion that there can be an objective description of a person's brain state or that the images can be used to predict future behavior. Does one violent reaction seen on brain imaging mean that, without intervention, the person will be a threat to society? The notion of biological determinism—in this case, that brain activity determines who you are and how you will behave—is troubling to many people. This is especially the case when the brain activity reveals socially negative responses or impulses. The studies described above and their conclusions also cause one to wonder what brain-imaging data mean to the individual, if and how the imaging will be used to control an identified social problem, and how we can find a judicious balance between the needs and rights of the individual and those of society in collecting, storing, and using neuroimaging data.

Another anticipated use of fMRI is to test the suitability of people for certain types of job. Dr. Moreno also commented on a study conducted at Emory University in which neuroimaging was used to distinguish people who like to cooperate from those who do not (Moreno 2003). The study showed that more women than men produced brain activity indicating pleasure (i.e., dopamine-rich neurons were activated) when they engaged in cooperative acts. Suppose, asked the ethicist, that businesses that value individually competitive employees want to use the Emory study to justify using fMRI as a screening device to eliminate cooperative people from the employment candidate pool? What if the company does not know whether the brain activity information adds anything significant to other screening devices, such as letters of recommendation or psychological testing? The author concludes by wondering about the reactions to the use: Will the scans be received as unacceptably invasive or just part of the job search routine?

While these kinds of questions were being posed, the adoption of fMRI technology leap-frogged straight into commercial territory with the founding of the
Brighthouse Institute for Thought Sciences in Atlanta. The institute describes
itself as the first neuromarketing research company with a vision "to help companies create better products, services and messages by providing them with un-
precedented insight about how to connect with their consumers." Neuromarketing studies were also being conducted at Emory University and the Mind of
the Market Laboratory at Harvard Business School. Companies such as General
Motors, Coca-Cola, Delta Air Lines, and MetLife started taking advantage of the
technology and paid for studies on consumers willing to undergo brain scanning
as they watched various company ads and images. Companies that used neuroimaging believed it was a better measure of marketing effectiveness because, in
essence, brain images don't lie and evidence of how the brain reacts is a more
accurate predictor of purchasing potential than what the consumer says (Wells
2003; Wahlberg 2004). Controversy about this application of neuroimaging was
quick in coming. Increasing the effectiveness of product advertising seemed a
dire prospect to many, especially those who sought to wean their children away
from its seductiveness. One critic pointed out that epidemics of obesity, diabetes,
alcoholism, gambling, smoking, and body-image problems were all tied to marketing and predicted that society will suffer if this activity increases. The scientists at the Brighthouse Institute and some outside researchers disagree and claim
that they are simply giving companies a way to better target their ad messages.
The fear that such ads will turn people into consumer automatons is overwrought,
they say. The brain is just not that simple, and people temper their emotional
reactions with judgment in deciding what to buy. According to a Dartmouth University associate professor of psychology, "It would be arrogant to say we could
stick someone in a machine and understand everything" (Wells 2003, p. 62).

THE CASE STUDY

It is the year 2008, and Dr. Jerome Golda is seeing the first person of the
day at the Cabeza Psychiatric Clinic, a private group practice that has been designed to bring multiple disciplines to the treatment of mental health problems.
Dr. Golda is a neuropsychiatrist; his colleagues include psychologists, transac-
tional analysts, radiologists, and pharmacologists. Modern psychiatric practice is
increasingly employing brain-imaging technologies to assist the more traditional
psychiatric methods to diagnose and treat mental illness. Accordingly, the clinic
has for some years had a state-of-the-art functional magnetic resonance imaging

facility, which is now often used in patient evaluation and in monitoring treatment. Because fMRI images produce what is believed to be objective understanding of how brain function affects or determines emotions, including tem-
perament, personality, and mood, Dr. Golda often relies on fMRI to tell him how
the brains of his patients are malfunctioning and whether various interventions
are restoring normal function.

The Patient

That is what is under way in Dr. Golda's examination of John Patton, an engaging and energetic 18-year-old who has been under treatment for symptoms
that have been disturbing John and his family. He is given to bouts of sudden, apparently inexplicable rage; these have not resulted in violence to others, but on
two recent occasions he has damaged objects—in one instance, destroying a television set following an upset loss by his favorite NFL team and in another case
smashing some expensive china during a family holiday gathering.

John had been diagnosed by his primary psychiatrist as having antisocial personality disorder. Before being referred to Dr. Golda, John had been seen for several sessions by a psychoanalyst, Dr. Hyde. John's family history is considered
pertinent to his current behavior in that he comes from a long line of military
officers, several of whom attended military schools and were early volunteers for
combat during times of war. The men in his family have a reputation for positive
aggressiveness, boldness, and leadership, but there is also some suggestion of a
tendency toward verbal (and possibly physical) abusiveness. When Dr. Hyde had
asked John about his childhood, he had found an unusual level of hostility about
John's treatment by his mother, apparently a very strict parent. John had volunteered that he rarely experienced uncontrollable anger during his frequent arguments with his mother. Dr. Hyde had also learned that, in his first year in high
school, John had begun to display fits of temper, to the extent that school authorities occasionally called his parents and once suspended him for a short time.
John has admitted that such episodes have become increasingly frequent in his
life, enough so to worry his family seriously.

With this information and assessment in hand, John was turned over to
Dr. Golda for an evaluation of the neurobiological basis for his emotional problems. Dr. Golda had already conducted MRI studies of the boy and found some
structural changes in the brain (smaller than normal intracranial and cerebral
volumes) that have been associated with post-traumatic stress disorder, possibly
resulting from past mistreatment at home. To assess any functional component

to John's behavior, Dr. Golda decided that it would be useful to create video scenarios for John to view while fMRI studies were being conducted, to perform fMRI studies during an interview with Dr. Hyde, and to combine these techniques in some sessions. The technical staff at Cabeza borrowed photographs of John's parents and others who were important in his childhood and used them to create computer-generated scenarios that can be played on a miniature TV screen fitted within the fMRI mount in the examination room while fMRI measurements are taken.

In one of these manufactured scenarios, the simulated video shows John's mother and father engaged in a disagreement so intense that his mother strikes his father, an incident that John had previously reported in detail to Dr. Hyde as one that had triggered what John characterized as typical of his anger reaction toward his mother. When John watches the scenario, he reports anger at his mother, and the fMRI study shows intense activity in an area of his brain (the amygdala) that is known to be involved in responding to and producing anger, avoidance, defensiveness, and fear. This neural reaction was expected, but what is troubling about the image is that the areas of the brain responsible for regulating anger responses (orbitofrontal cortices) do not "light up" appropriately. Together, these findings suggest that young Patton has functional brain patterns that predispose him to react strongly to anger stimuli with a diminished ability to control his behavior in response to anger. John is therefore considered to be at high risk for violent behavior in the future. While this kind of prognosis had been made in the past, it had typically been imprecise, based only on traditional psychiatric evaluations and behavior tests. Studies have shown that obtaining consistent fMRI data greatly enhances the confidence with which such a prognosis can be made.

1. Is this technique of provoking a reaction so it can be imaged justified? Is it ethical? Would this evaluation scenario, had it been done in the research setting, required IRB approval? What validation standards should exist for this kind of diagnostic use of neuroimaging?

2. What standards should be in place before fMRI is used to diagnose behavior disorders? Who should be involved in developing them?

3. If patients know in advance that such scenarios will be presented, some will be able to modify their reactions to them, so Dr. Golda avoids giving patients a precise advance description of the assessment scenarios. In clinical practice, how should a psychiatrist obtain consent for this kind of assessment? Should warnings be required?

4. Did the psychiatrist have obligations to inform or get permission from John's parents before creating a video that "reinvents" their past and puts them in a negative light?

What If We Can Diagnose but Can't Treat?

Although researchers and pharmaceutical company scientists have translated MRI and fMRI information about different brain structure and circuitry into new treatments for panic disorder and anxiety syndromes, there is as yet no proven therapy to help young Patton. No treatments are available that can moderate the abnormal brain responses to anger that are triggered by neural activity in the amygdala and orbitofrontal cortex. In addition, anger-management therapy has been only inconsistently effective in the type of neural reactions seen here. The findings and lack of treatment options all lead to the conclusion that John will exhibit an increasing tendency to react angrily to less provocative stimuli. As a consequence, although the neural findings are not completely determinative, the physicians are fairly certain that John's abnormal behavior will continue and worsen over time.

5. What should John be told about his brain-imaging studies and what they indicate?

6. What are the likely consequences of patients' being told that their brain works in ways that will make them destructive? What are the implications of thinking that brain physiology is responsible for aberrant behavior rather than perceiving behavior as something controlled by the will? Should we hold these people completely responsible for their actions, given that they appear to be at a physiological disadvantage?

7. Would it be legitimate to use neural imaging to classify people as aggressive or nonaggressive? What positive and negative uses could be made of such a classification?

8. What are the implications of classifying as medical conditions (here, aggressiveness) states that were previously attributed primarily to social influences?

9. Would the power of functional brain imaging justify requiring John's mental health caregivers to warn people who would closely associate with him?

10. What conditions should exist to justify functional neuroimaging in people who have not exhibited mental health or behavioral problems? If the

imaging is powerfully predictive of behavior, can it be used to sort people for characteristics such as aptitude? If so, what consequences might flow from this use? And who is entitled to this information?

What If We Can Treat?

Later, some neurosurgeons develop what is believed to be a very precise way to create a lesion in the brain exactly where it will dampen the reaction to anger stimuli. John Patton's psychiatrist wonders whether he is a candidate for the procedure. He is now 31 years old and has been arrested once for violent behavior. Also in the offing is a drug that can be used to enhance the ability of the brain to modulate aggression.

11. Would it be appropriate to treat John Patton with these therapies? What are legitimate bases for making the choice between them?

12. Does the precision with which fMRI can monitor the physiological responses to these therapies make them potentially better than existing brain stimulators or drugs that control behavior?

13. At what point does the use of such therapies become a disturbing form of social control? Might there be a tendency, even if behavior is similar, to recommend the new treatments more readily for patients from lower social classes than for a young man from a family of distinguished military officers such as the Pattons?

14. How much aberration is needed to justify employing these therapies, and how much alteration in mental function can be justified, especially if the alteration changes personality or changes how people experience life?

The Law Becomes Involved

While in his twenties, John Patton was involved in an abusive incident, in which his girlfriend sustained injuries sufficient to require emergency care. This incident was seemingly unprovoked (or provoked by very little) and was consistent with the psychiatric and biological prognosis that Patton was at risk for this type of behavior. The district attorney of Patton's jurisdiction, having read the police report and the warrant for Patton's arrest, decided to prosecute him for assault and battery. In the course of the legal proceeding, Patton's attorney asks that the records of his treatment, including the fMRI images, be introduced as exculpatory evidence in his behalf.

15. What do we think about the use of biological evidence (genotype, brain images, etc.) as exculpatory evidence in a criminal matter? Should people be held completely responsible for their actions, even if they appear to be at a physiological disadvantage? How should the personal autonomy of people like John Patton be balanced against public safety?

16. If fMRI evidence can be exculpatory, are all prisoners entitled to brain scans as part of their defense?

17. A proposed amendment to Great Britain's Mental Health Act would allow the detention of individuals who have not yet committed a crime but are deemed a potential threat to public safety. Would preventive detention be a reasonable response to learning that persons' brain functions predispose them to violence? Should people with abnormal brain images be reported to law enforcement authorities? The U.S. Supreme Court has ruled that violent sex offenders can be jailed beyond their prison term if it can be shown that they have a mental or personality disorder that makes it difficult for them to control dangerous behavior. How can fMRI be used constructively in such complex situations?

CHAPTER SEVEN

Questions, Issues, and Recommendations Going Forward

Many people believe that innovators are medicine's heroes—men and women who are not resigned in the face of impending death or disability but instead look for ways to improve treatment options for their patients. Many patients have benefited from the boldness of countless physicians who have innovated on their behalf. Physicians who succeed as innovators are often esteemed by their peers, and they reap justifiable professional and personal rewards for their achievements. Given all of these benefits, it is not surprising that some physicians believe they have a duty to innovate and should be accorded the freedom to do so as a professional prerogative.

On the other hand, despite its benefits, medical innovation deployed outside of a research environment often occurs haphazardly and may be implemented without producing generally useable data regarding the consequences. Ideally, medical innovations originate from a sound theoretical base, but some are also supported by little more than hopeful guesswork. Empiricism also supports the development of new treatments, which again can be solid or based only on the fact that a treatment seems to work, without an understanding of how or why it works. This lack of consistency or standard practice in how innovations come about has led to recommendations that most medical innovation should be subject to research requirements. Rather than relying on trial and error, the argument goes, carefully controlled and executed studies will produce the most reliable information about the benefits and risks of new therapies and procedures. Innovation based on research allows physicians to move beyond inference to a greater certainty (depending on the trustworthiness of the data) that a treatment or practice is beneficial.

These divergent views were discussed at the Lasker Foundation Forum that led to this book. The forum's participants identified four core questions and issues that should guide any consideration of how new medical technologies should be deployed.

1. Should medical innovation be deployed as research or as medical practice?
2. What are the thresholds and models for oversight?
3. What information should be disclosed to patients?
4. Is there a professional duty to learn and to educate other practitioners?

SHOULD MEDICAL INNOVATION BE DEPLOYED AS MEDICAL RESEARCH OR AS MEDICAL PRACTICE?

All of those who have addressed this question have faced the difficulty of distinguishing between medical research and medical practice. Despite their seeming differences, the dividing line can be hard to find. The distinction can depend on the context in which an innovation takes place. For instance, a change in surgical technique intended to reduce the chance of cutting a nerve seems more like adaptive practice and unlike using a drug for a disease for the first time, which seems more like research. But there are many times when it is difficult to distinguish between changes that should be researched before general implementation and changes that are merely innovation "creep," where physicians are changing therapy or technique to fit the needs of patients.

Despite its attempt at clarification, the Belmont Report leaves many questions on the distinction between research and practice open for further discussion. Much research is conducted with a reasonable belief that human subjects will benefit medically, and plenty of physicians and surgeons would disagree about what constitutes a "radical" departure from standard practice and thus requires a research protocol. Because change in medical practice is often characterized by a continuous stream of small innovations, the attendant incremental progress crosses no bright line into agreed definitions of formal research. So how is one to distinguish between the two? Despite a professional and academic dialogue that began more than thirty years ago in the United States, there still seems to be no consistent opinion.

The range of views on the subject is typified by the account relayed by a surgeon at the Lasker Forum. He described an innovative practice that resulted when a colleague attempted to improve the postoperative results of balloon angioplasty followed by the insertion of a coronary stent.[1] Surgeons generally had been in favor of using the stents but were frustrated by the fact that stent patients experienced an unacceptably high rate of potentially fatal blood clots, despite the use of a blood thinner, warfarin. Although it was counterintuitive, this particular surgeon suspected that the blood thinner was actually causing the blood clots. He also had ultrasound evidence that placing the stents using conventional balloon pressures was leaving the stent inadequately expanded, which might also cause clotting. The combination of the surgeon's suspicion about the drug and his ultrasound evidence led him to start performing the angioplasty procedure using higher balloon pressures and withholding the postoperative warfarin. Despite the fear that these changes would both damage the artery from excessive pressure and increase postoperative blood clotting, the changes succeeded and have now become standard practice. According to the physician relaying this story, it was a "brave experiment" that "made a huge difference in the way we now practice." Some who heard the story called it "gutsy," while others shuddered at the risk that was taken. A similar range of views existed among the Lasker Forum participants who discussed the surgery case study presented in Chapter 4 of this book.

When a physician adopts a procedure well beyond the standard of care, it is clearly difficult to tell whether the action will bring about an advance in that standard. In the angioplasty surgery case just described, no formal research preceded the "brave experiment" that worked. Surgeons, especially, often assume that formal research is not needed prior to use of a new technique, because operative observation alone will disclose whether the innovation works as intended. This is not always the case, however, because the long-term effects of new surgical techniques (e.g., blood clots, failed repairs, need for repeat surgeries) can often be assessed only by systematically comparing the innovation with the standard method or placebo surgery. With medical innovations, it is more commonly believed that benefits and risks will not be fully understood until formal research is conducted. Yet, many standard medical practices have not been subjected to controlled research, a situation which leaves physicians practicing in an environment of either perpetual uncertainty or unfounded certainty. A recent example involved the first controlled study, published in 2002, of the use of postmenopausal hormone replacement therapy (HRT). For decades, HRT had been prescribed long term to postmenopausal women, in the belief (supported primarily by anecdotal evidence or uncontrolled studies) that this therapy prevented or delayed cardiovascular disease, bone thinning, and other common diseases associated with aging in women. Not only did the new study fail to support many of the beneficial claims for HRT, it showed that the therapy was associated with an increase of breast cancer, heart attack, stroke, and blood clots in the lungs (pulmonary embolism) and legs (deep venous thrombosis) (Writing Group for the Women's Health Initiative Investigators 2002). Earlier research clearly would have led to more informed prescribing practices.

Other benefits of conducting research on medical innovations include that patients enrolled in studies are afforded specific consent rights and that study protocols are reviewed in advance by an institution's IRB, which seeks to ensure that the risks to participants are reasonable in relation to expected benefits and that participants are chosen equitably. No such standards exist for nonresearch innovation.

But, if all innovation were subject to research requirements, would medicine and surgery have advanced as they have in the United States? For instance, according to one participant in the assisted reproductive technology discussion group at the Lasker Forum, "If you have to wait until the child is of mature age before deciding if the culture medium works, you'll be paralyzed." Outside of research, innovations are tailored to individual patient needs, worthwhile medical innovations tend to be implemented much faster, and harmful innovations can be rejected sooner. Research, on the other hand, often involves delay, high costs, multiple personnel, and administrative burdens. At its most formal, medical research requires preparing and submitting a study protocol to an IRB, waiting for approval (often months in coming), enrolling large numbers of human subjects in a lengthy study, rigorously managing the conduct of the study, and then statistically analyzing the results and reporting them. Other physicians challenge the notion that research necessarily burdens and limits innovation. The assumption, they say, that research requirements slow down innovation is just that—an assumption—and should be tested. IRB and research processes might speed and benefit innovation, by proving earlier knowledge about which treatments and procedures are beneficial and which are not. And besides, as the HRT study exemplifies, even research that takes time might be well worth the wait.

However, research does not always remove the uncertainty associated with innovation that occurs within medical practice. The colloquy that follows the publication of research findings indicates that it is sometimes difficult to make supportable conclusions from the data. Some research deficiencies stem from careless or intentional mismanagement, other problems are inherent in the nature of human research. For one thing, research physicians with greater experience will likely have better results with new technologies than physicians with less experience, so exactly who executed the study can affect the results. Close scrutiny of the details of clinical research sometimes shows that protocol design has skewed the study results, that subject selection was not rigorous enough, that the principal investigator assigned research duties to insufficiently trained junior staff, that data was inconsistently analyzed or, on rare occasions, invented (Pocock et al. 2004; White 2005). Large trials performed at multiple centers can suffer from inconsistencies in protocol implementation. Some medical disciplines are more prone to these difficulties than are others. Psychiatrists, for instance, can often disagree on a patient's diagnosis, which introduces a significant variation in subject selection into large psychiatric drug trials. Conflicts of interest can also undermine the validity of research findings, a situation exemplified by the findings that drug trials sponsored by pharmaceutical companies report positive results more often than do drug trials under different sponsorship (Stelfox et al. 1998). Intratrial problems such as these, which make data interpretation difficult, are magnified when one tries to compare studies purporting to assess the same medical technology but which arrived at different conclusions. In addition, attempting to determine the efficacy and safety of new treatments can be confounded because positive results tend to be published more often than negative ones, researchers sometimes publish the same study more than once, and some poorly designed studies can get published despite careful peer review by journal editors and expert reviewers (Rennie 1999). Because it is a human endeavor, there will always be a certain amount of these kinds of sloppiness associated with clinical research.

In the application of research results to practice, an inherent limitation is that research findings are applicable only to patients with the same characteristics as the subjects who were studied. For instance, although the HRT study has been viewed as applying to postmenopausal women in general, the study results are probably applicable only to women similar to the study population (women who started taking estrogen 10–15 years after the onset of menopause) and not to younger women who start taking HRT at the onset of menopause. Research findings also apply only for as long as the research was conducted. Therefore, a two-year drug trial does not inform about the consequences of taking the drug for four years. Data also cannot be extrapolated. For example, even though the point of taking an anticancer drug is to extend life, a study showing that a drug slows the rate of tumor progression is not sufficient to make a valid claim that it extends life. Despite the recognized benefits, therefore, research cannot always mitigate the deficiencies of deploying innovations in a practice setting.

As there are different views about the benefits of research, there are also disagreements on the related question of whether medical innovation should be regulated. The history of IVF is instructive in this regard. According to many reports, it was common for the first U.S. physician groups who performed IVF to experience up to 100 failures within a practice and to persist for ten years before achieving their first successful pregnancy. It typically took two years after that for the first pregnancy to be carried full term and successfully delivered. Then, from 1978 to 1998, success rates rose progressively, a result of incremental changes in IVF methodology that permitted more cycles, more implantations, and more births. According to critics of requiring controlled testing, if every IVF change had been subjected to regulation and research, these successes would have occurred much more slowly and resulted in fewer births. This opinion is supported by statistics kept by the American Society of Reproductive Medicine (ASRM) which show that there are definite differences in IVF outcomes in regulated versus non-regulated environments. In the unregulated United States, IVF now results in a 35 percent birth rate. In the regulated environment of the United Kingdom, where the number of implanted embryos is limited, the birth rate is closer to 18 percent. However, the percentage of single births (the preferred result) in the United States is 65 percent versus the U.K. rate of 78 percent. In the United States, twins (somewhat risky) are produced at a rate of 31 percent compared to the U.K. rate of 20 percent, and giving birth to three or more children (fairly dangerous) occurs at a rate of 3–4 percent in the United States, whereas in the United Kingdom, the rate is between 2 and 3 percent. Even allowing for the suspicion that there is a tendency in the United States to report overly favorable data, these are significant differences.[2] With findings like these, it is easy to see why disagreement exists on whether a regulated or nonregulated system is better.

Despite the different views about the way medical innovation should proceed, there are areas of agreement on the research versus practice issue. One concerns the utility of the definition of research according to the FDA and the DHHS.[3] Most commentators (including the participants at the Lasker Forum) feel that these definitions are not helpful in deciding whether medical or surgical innovations should proceed as advanced practice or should require IRB approval under a research protocol. In the Common Rule definition of research, the intent of the physician is key in deciding whether he or she is engaging in research. But the prevailing view is that examining physician intent is not the best way to reach such a conclusion. Innovating physicians usually have multiple intentions; they want to help a particular patient, but they also want to advance the state of the art and produce knowledge for the benefit of future patients. Physicians may also intend to improve their own careers by publishing or becoming a resource for a certain novel treatment or procedure. Most of the time, these multiple intentions are sincerely held and compatible. But, intent is unobservable and subject to manipulation. A distinction that depends upon the physician's motive makes it attractive for physicians who lack access to a research infrastructure or who want to avoid the restrictions and requirements of research to declare that their primary intent is treatment, not research. Another problem with using intent to distinguish research is that some physicians formulate an intent to contribute to generalizable knowledge after the fact, for example, after discovering how successful a procedural adaptation was. A physician's retrospective publication of outcome data on a new treatment might be viewed as an improper end-run around an IRB approval requirement, which could subject the physician to discipline. This conclusion often is unfair, because it effectively punishes a physician who may have only intended to share valuable information about a treatment improvement.

Another area of agreement concerns a physician's degree of confidence about the prospects of success of a medical innovation. The relevance of this factor in deciding whether the innovation should be subject to research should not be underestimated. Innovating physicians as a class are remarkably self-confident professionals, a quality that enhances their effectiveness, because self-confidence is often required to take the risks necessary to push the medical technology envelope. The physician's confidence also often spills over to the patient and promotes trust and compliance. The subjective belief by a physician that a new technique is beneficial, however, may be suspect in many cases. The problem with self-confidence is that it can become overconfidence and can cause physicians to lose objectivity. But, if the physician-innovator is not the one who decides whether the new aspect of practice requires research, there is no uniform agreement about who should be. Do IRBs do a better job at making the distinction between research and innovative practice? Many physicians find that seeking an advisory opinion from an IRB automatically results in a finding that the activity falls within the IRB's jurisdiction and constitutes research.

These many questions are continuously debated in the medical profession, and there is currently no satisfactory uniform approach to the question of research versus treatment. There are guidelines (such as from the Belmont Report) for what constitutes research, and physicians routinely adapt the general guidelines to individual patients and their own personal preferences and intuitions. This subjective adaptation contributes to disagreement over whether innovation should be subject to regulation and if so what kind, making it very difficult to decide how best to manage innovation without stifling progress and effectively countenancing irresponsible experimentation disguised as treatment.

Overall, the existing binary choice between research and practice is probably too constraining, because, given the current rapid pace of innovation, too much of medical and surgical innovation seems to fall in the middle of the spectrum.

Many new procedures and techniques are performed both to produce knowledge and to assist the patient. If this is how the real world works, then the system should acknowledge it and be adapted. It seems prudent, therefore, to create a category to accommodate this kind of intermediate situation, even if solely to make explicit what the physician is doing. Alternative terminology could trigger a mindfulness in the practitioner that he or she is engaged in something that has aspects of both treatment and research. Some of the Belmont commentators used the term *innovative therapy*. Suggestions from Lasker Forum participants for additions to the lexicon included: *crossover therapy, unproved therapy, nonvalidated intervention, exploratory practice, clinical innovation,* and *pilot innovation.* Regardless of what innovative activities are called, it seems better to reclassify them than to force them into the current (and sometimes arbitrary) definitions and parameters of either research or medical practice.

With this as a starting point, we can move on to tackle the questions inspired by recognizing that innovation is taking place: Does the deviation from standard medical care rise to a level of ethical significance that should require oversight or research? Are there specific disclosures that should be made to patients? Is there a professional duty to learn more and educate others about the impact of the innovation on patients?

WHAT ARE THE THRESHOLDS AND MODELS FOR OVERSIGHT?

If medical innovation does not fit within the traditional rubric of either research (with oversight provided by an IRB or a regulatory agency such as the FDA) or medical practice (generally free from oversight except when the physician's career is reviewed before the granting of hospital admitting privileges or when a complaint is lodged with the hospital or the state licensing board), how can oversight be provided, to ensure that innovation is deployed in a responsible fashion? In responding to this question, one needs to determine the threshold criteria that would trigger a need for oversight and to identify models of systems that can provide appropriate oversight.

Considering all of the stakeholders' interests, the goals of any oversight should include the protection of patients, the promotion of high medical practice standards, and the preservation of trust in medical practice and research. Therefore, thresholds for oversight might be found by focusing on the patient, the physician, the setting, and the broader context. Focusing on the patient, it seems prudent to favor oversight when the innovation represents a significant deviation from standard medical practice, when the potential risk for lack of efficacy or risk of harm from the treatment or procedure is high, and when there is insufficient evidence to support the adoption of the innovation into practice. Focusing on the physician, triggers for oversight should include treatments in which the physician has a research intent (meaning the physician intends to collect and disseminate data), in which patient care competes with other interests of the physician, and in which significant retraining is required to provide the treatment. The triggers that focus on the setting should include whether the hospital is known for its research orientation or use of innovative technologies and has the expertise and resources to support these activities. Triggers relating to the broader context include ethical, economic, and social factors such as whether there are any significant financial or other conflicts of interest at play and whether there are any third-party interests involved, such as the children born of assisted reproductive technology or nonmedical personnel who might seek neuroimaging findings. As with all past attempts to find dividing lines in this field, there will be differences of opinion in what is "significant" when considering deviations from standard care, physician retraining, conflicts of interest, and so forth. These differences seem unavoidable, in part because physicians and institutions practice medicine and surgery at different levels of expertise. As a result, internal conceptions of what constitutes significance in these matters most likely correlate with the level of medical practice, and this is probably appropriate. What is perhaps more important is that these questions be addressed, so that innovation does not proceed without some consideration of whether oversight would be advisable.

Regarding appropriate models, one might ask whether medical innovation oversight should be based on models used by state licensing agencies (which have a consumer protection focus or mandate reporting of certain events), hospital medical staffs (which credential and rely on peer review), professional societies (which use practice guidelines or form consortia to engage in cooperative activities), government agencies (which promulgate regulations, such as those pertaining to human subject protection), or those systems that depend on incentives or disincentives (e.g., funding versus medical malpractice liability).

Physicians tend to favor oversight only if it comes from the relevant medical profession. In this view, government or other bureaucratic oversight is too burdensome, at least for the early stages of innovation, given the rapidity with which medicine is advancing. Professional oversight can be speedy and flexible and conducted by experts who understand the capabilities and limits of the technology. Medical professionals can also achieve scientific and medical agreement, which should always exist before laws governing technology and medical practice are put into place. All of these factors make professional oversight preferable. Others favor oversight and advice on innovation from an interdisciplinary advisory structure with broader goals, such as empowering investigators and clinicians, protecting patients, and promoting public trust in the use of the technology. One entity that has put this oversight model into practice is the Massachusetts General Hospital Innovative Diagnostics and Therapeutics Committee. This committee, composed of members from many relevant disciplines, was formed to review new medical technologies (diagnostics, drugs, and procedures) and determine the circumstances under which they should be deployed.[4] The committee provides guidance and support to physicians unsure about whether their new treatments should undergo research examination or can be implemented as practice without it (and, if so, under what circumstances). The technology that stimulated the formation of the committee and serves as an example of how medical technology can be introduced without a formal research process is a form of continuous hemodialysis called continuous venovenous hemofiltration (CVVH). The new technology was developed to treat critically ill patients with renal failure who, because they were too unstable, could not be treated with conventional intermittent dialysis. The hospital committee provided useful guidance and advice as this technology was introduced into patient care. CVVH now significantly increases the survival rate of such patients with acute renal failure.[5] The Massachusetts General committee has gone on to review three or four significant technologies annually, and it shepherds and monitors the ones it endorses.

Another more formal and widespread technology assessment program that might also serve as a template exists at the U.S. Agency for Healthcare Research and Quality (AHRQ), which evaluates the safety and effectiveness of new or as-yet-unproven medical technologies and procedures that are being considered for coverage under Medicare and Medicaid. AHRQ technology assessments are based on a systematic review of the medical literature, along with appropriate qualitative and quantitative syntheses of data from multiple studies. Technology assessments may be done in-house by AHRQ staff, or they may be done in collaboration with one of its twelve Evidence-based Practice Centers, which have evaluated such medical technologies as the use if islet cell transplantation for diabetes, testosterone suppression treatment for prostatic cancer, and hyperbaric oxygen treatment of brain injuries and stroke.[6]

Since the formation of these two new oversight bodies, some writers on the subject have advocated similar peer or stakeholder review committees to provide a form of oversight less burdensome than the existent IRB processes and to do assessment of treatments and procedures where professional uncertainty exists (McKneally and Daar 2003). Proposals for these oversight and assessment committees most often assume that dual purposes can be accommodated in their function—promoting innovation while assuring the safety and efficacy of new medical treatments. Also, proponents have advocated both local committees (similar to the Massachusetts General committee) or national entities. If a national body is desired, private professional societies (so long as they remained impartial) or organizations such as the Institute of Medicine could fulfill the role. While this task could also be assigned to a new governmental body, assumptions about the inevitable bureaucracy make this the least favored choice. If the AHRQ took on the job, it would have to be reconfigured to include the assessment of technologies that have not generated research data. There is doubt about the extent to which funding would be available for an additional governmental oversight entity. Other more general doubts about oversight and assessment committees include the risk that, if a committee was dominated by fellow (i.e., knowledgeable) practitioners, it could become an exercise in rubber stamping. Also, review committees might generate administrative and procedural requirements that would mimic and become as burdensome as an IRB process. Finally, any committee is likely to have problems in accommodating both patient safety and innovation support goals.

Regardless of the particular method or process, most commentators and the Lasker group agree that some sort of oversight, advice, and approval should be required for particular medical innovations before offering the treatment to patients. These innovations would include only those most "obviously" in need of guidance, which is to say, there should be a high bar to distinguish those innovations that require oversight. Otherwise, oversight of innovation could become the regulation of most medical care. One major caveat, however, is that before any oversight scheme is put into place, the medical community must be convinced that the harms or problems engendered by medical innovation are of a sufficient magnitude to justify the burdens of oversight. Once this is established— granted, not a simple matter—any oversight should address the specific risks, be workable, should use existing resources, should not reinvent the wheel (i.e., should adopt other programs that have worked, such as payor criteria used to classify reimbursable medical treatments), and help the innovator as much as possible with as little burden as possible. In addition, local and national resources should be used only for what they do best; forcing entities to change their focus or adopt different responsibilities would not be a workable solution. Finally, any oversight program should also have a mechanism to disseminate outcome information about new treatments.

WHAT INFORMATION SHOULD BE DISCLOSED TO PATIENTS?

Because meaningful oversight does not exist for much of medical innovation that is deployed as medical practice (and sometimes even when it is researched first), disclosure about treatment risks and benefits is fundamental to protecting patient interests. In the experience of those who have studied the issue, disclosure practices vary widely. For instance, in one Canadian study of patient brochures used in IVF clinics, disclosures seemed more confusing than enlightening: the study found that the patient information brochures were written at a postgraduate level of education and were not comprehensible to the average person. IVF success rates were defined in twelve or fifteen different ways and were found to be misleading. It is clear that the written information reviewed in this study was inadequate. Deciding what constitutes adequate disclosure, however, is a difficult task. And this difficulty is increased by the rapidity with which practices change and the relative paucity of available data about innovative treatments, especially about the long-term consequences.

There is general agreement that some basic guidelines should be used to determine what information to disclose about innovative treatments. Generally, patients need enough information about proposed treatments to allow them to exercise their right to make autonomous decisions regarding whether or not to participate. Respecting autonomy requires that full information (as much as can be known) be provided in circumstances free from undue influence or coercion. Predictions about the benefits of medical technology should not be made without a reasonable expectation that they can be fulfilled. Also, disclosures should not always be limited to the medical consequences of treatment. If treatment can negatively impact the patient psychically or socially, this should be disclosed, especially with predictive interventions (which can reveal a predisposition for a particular disease) that can have impacts such as the loss of employment or insurance, the loss of medical privacy, and stigmatization. Generally, disclosures should increase in correlation to the degree of uncertainty about the outcome of a procedure. As with all things ethical, motive matters; and patient disclosures should not be motivated by physician self-interest, for instance, to avoid litigation. Such a motivation often provides the patient with an extensive litany of possible risks that does not assist the patient in making meaningful choices.

Patients also need information for emotional reasons, because knowing in advance about the probabilities of treatment failure or harm can mitigate feelings of guilt, anger, despair, or betrayal that patients experience when things go wrong. The consent process can also address other emotional aspects of treatment, such as patients' need to trust their doctor and to have hope when few treatment options exist. For example, one oncologist might tell a patient that he is recommending a "mouse" procedure, because the procedure has so far been used mostly on mice but has been successful in very few humans. Or, in the same situation, another physician might say that he is there to help the patient in any way he can and that the procedure offers a chance of getting the patient out of the woods. Both disclosures are accurate. The first is maximally candid and eliminates false expectations but may make the physician appear callous and may cause a patient to reject the last remaining treatment option. The second is optimistic, communicates commitment, and allows the patient to hope, which can be therapeutic; but it also deemphasizes the risks and allows positive inferences that may not be justified. It takes a sensitive physician to convey pessimistic information with balance and candor without destroying hope.

Appreciation for patients' emotional vulnerability in the medical treatment process leads to consideration of how innovative treatment information should be given so that it is not overly persuasive or optimistic. Most physicians are aware that surgeons typically have an enormous influence on what procedures patients will consent to. According to one Lasker Forum participant, when the surgeon is very famous, some patients "will leap at the chance to have the surgery done by him, even to be the first patient. They say, 'I'd be anything (patient or research subject) so long as this man can do my surgery.'" A senior surgeon in the group said, "I have never had a patient refuse to undergo a surgery that I recommended and I find this terrifying." Another surgeon participant cited a 1922 medical journal article entitled "The Physician as Placebo" and commented "Our placebo effect starts at the time a patient starts talking with us. The process is extraordinary." Yet another participant told a story to emphasize the point that the influence of a physician is universal and applies even to other sophisticated physicians when they become patients: A nationally famous and influential Boston physician developed cancer and sought the advice of as many physicians as he could. However, he became deeply conflicted about which of the many and varied treatment options to accept. A colleague suggested he "stop obsessing" about treatment options and instead pick one doctor he trusted, just one. The physician did just that, consented to the recommended treatment, and reported that he right away felt much better about his situation. As with many patients, it was not weighing the benefits and risks of the treatments that persuaded him to consent; it was his trust in his physician that was the deciding factor.

Given their persuasive influence, the power physicians wield in the consent process needs to be explicitly recognized and tempered. One Lasker Forum participant commented that she was more concerned about the manner in which Dr. Oldwest in the assisted reproductive technology case managed the consent process than she was about how he had tinkered with the embryo culture medium. This participant felt that Dr. O came across as imposing his decisions on the patient (the number of embryos to implant, genetic diagnosis, etc.) rather than soliciting the patient's views after a calm and thorough discussion. There was doubt among some other participants about whether most physicians recommending their own innovative treatments would be as aggressive as Dr. O in the consent process. Certainly, doctors should be confident about what they recommend for patients, but the degree to which most physicians translate confidence into an imposition of will is debated. It has been suggested that an overly confident physician, especially one who stands to gain financially through the use of his own inventions, should perhaps allow the disclosure process to be done by someone else. A disinterested third-party counselor would focus on disclosure and comprehension and act as an objective decision-making guide. This suggestion appeals to those who believe that most physicians are interested in the medical treatment and give short shrift to the consent process because they find it uninteresting. But, implementing a consent process using a third party introduces several difficulties. Two significant problems were identified, in addition to those of privacy, logistics, and cost: (1) patients most often want to speak directly with the physician who will provide the treatment, and (2) it may not be good policy to allow physicians to assign to others such a vital aspect of treatment.

Discussion of disclosure leads to the consideration of its intricate connection to decision making. In the best circumstances, full disclosure allows patients to make optimal decisions for themselves based on their personal values and preferences. However, this "doctor discloses/patient decides" model of consent may fail due to the confusing complexities of many new medical technologies or the patient's intellectual or emotional inability to comprehend the consequences of all the decisions that must be made. It is possible to present too much information. Suggestions have been made to address this dilemma. One is to have physicians ask patients how much detail they want and to tailor the disclosure to the expressed preference of the patient, but often patients are unable to say in advance what information is important to them and they simply defer to the doctor. Others, such as the Boston physician-patient, select their treatment by choosing a physician they trust and accepting whatever treatment is recommended. If a patient's primary care physician has recommended a specialist to that patient, the referral carries weight, and a climate of confidence in the new doctor is already established; it is a "referral and an anointment" that inclines the patient to consent to the specialist's recommendations.

Regardless of how actively patients participate in decision making, disclosure of the benefits and risks of treatment is a fundamental aspect of medical care. Yet, despite the importance of disclosure, there are times when it has little effect on the patient's choices. Physicians report that it is common for patients to listen to a description of the proposed treatment and then ask, "What would you do if you were in my shoes?" or "What if I was your mother; is this what you would recommend?" The answer to the question determines the patient's choice. Most physicians have also seen patients who are determined to proceed with a new intervention no matter how much risk information they are given in a consent discussion. These are motivated and passionate people; many are attempting to make life-altering decisions. Patients, especially those who have cancer or who are seeking care for a child, come to major academic medical centers expecting the latest innovations and they can be especially aggressive about obtaining treatment. Patients can be so desperate that they will consent to any treatment option no matter how untested or risky. Sometimes the desperation and hope overpower even the most thorough and conscientious attempts to provide for a well-informed consent.

Two recent incidents of this phenomenon are frequently mentioned, one involving fetal surgery for spina bifida and the other the use of monoclonal antibodies to treat brain cancer. Information about these two incidents provides some insight into the mix of influences that can induce a patient to demand innovative treatments despite the unknown risks.

Fetal surgery to correct spina bifida[7] was attempted in the late 1990s because conventional treatment, a series of postnatal surgical repairs, was often only minimally successful and left infants severely disabled. These problems led surgeons at Vanderbilt University Medical Center to test in utero corrections in animals and then to perform the first such surgeries on humans under an IRB-approved research protocol (Bruner et al. 1999).[8] As soon as a prominent medical journal published the first four case results (two infants survived with mild neurologic deficits, but the other two died), parents began to seek out this surgery. Then the lay press picked up the story. *Time* magazine's story used a cover picture of the tiny hand of a 21-week-old fetus clutching the gloved finger of a Vanderbilt surgeon, as if in a tiny plea for help. Immediately, desperate pregnant women around the country diagnosed as carrying spina bifida fetuses flocked to the two centers performing the procedure. Surgeons known to some of the Lasker Forum participants reported a 99 percent consent rate for the procedure, despite the fact that the procedure entailed significant (including lethal) risks—not only to the babies but to the women—and even when the surgeons told the parents that they were unsure if the benefits outweighed the risks (Tulipan et al. 2003).[9] But, one Lasker Forum participant asked, "What woman would refuse when the surgeon says 'I believe there is a chance we can help your baby'?"[10]

The other widely discussed incident occurred in 2000 at Duke University Medical Center and was featured on CBS's *48 Hours* television show. The episode described a patient who had been disease free four years after receiving an experimental monoclonal antibody cancer drug to treat a brain tumor that had been diagnosed previously as lethal and untreatable. In 2002, CBS's *60 Minutes* reported on the same Duke University physicians and the remarkable work they had done in saving the lives of some brain cancer victims with such experimental treatments. According to a Lasker Forum participant, these shows were "almost an ad for Duke Hospital" and prompted thousands of cancer patients to call the Duke center in the days following these broadcasts.[11] This patient reaction was not surprising, given the story told by the cancer survivor in the first broadcast. He was a young father who, determined to fight to the last, found the Duke center on the Internet, when looking for a doctor who was "out there rattling the cages, saying, 'We're going to save this guy'" (Battling a Brain Tumor 2000). The oncologist who did just that was the kind of pioneer physician determined to give patients every chance. He was quoted in the second television broadcast as saying that treatment must begin with hope. "We give them the motto that we stand by, which is 'at Duke, there is hope.' You can see almost a swelling within as the fight in them begins to resume, because they have been told before that it's absolutely, unequivocally hopeless, and without hope, it just ends before it begins" (Desperately Fighting Cancer 2002).

Views on these cases differ. Some will be resigned and believe that there was no way to avoid the automatic consent that results from a determined, despairing patient seeking treatment from a boldly innovative and confident physician. Some will deplore the fact that the consent process in such cases can turn into nothing more than a ritualistic formality, whereas others are prone to think that if patients want to take risky chances in an attempt to save their lives, they should be allowed to. Perhaps the consent process cannot be made to do something impossible, to throw the cold water of rationality and reason onto desperate circumstances.

Because of the myriad influences that undermine free and fully informed patient consent, one view holds that disclosure of all risks and benefits should not be viewed as a panacea and that physicians should sometimes not leave decisions up to the patient. Medical treatment information is becoming so complicated and access to this information is in so much flux that patients may have more facts but not more understanding. Because of this, it is said that patients now have both more and less ability to exercise autonomy in a medical relationship with their physicians. Consequently, there may still be a role for paternalism in medicine, an aspect of the profession that, although currently disfavored, can sometimes be justified. One participant in the assisted reproductive technology case study group suggested that there are some treatment decisions that physicians should make, such as when the physician, thinking of the child, determines that a risk of birth defect is too high even for a couple who would choose to go forward with implanting the embryo. There are also circumstances, such as when it is unlikely that a patient will experience any benefit, in which physicians should exercise ultimate control and refuse to provide innovative treatments, whatever the demands from patients. Despite the wisdom that physicians can bring to the consent process, however, cutting the patient out of the decision-making process is a dicey proposition in today's world, where patient autonomy is so highly valued.

Recognizing all of these obstacles to obtaining meaningful consent, one Lasker Forum subgroup developed the following list of recommendations about disclosing information to a patient about innovative treatments and procedures.

What to Disclose

- What a reasonable patient needs to know to make an informed choice, with the basics being the risks, benefits, and alternatives to any contemplated treatment
- Any conflict of interest
- Experiential status and realistic opinion about outcomes
- If the treatment is being provided in nonstandard ways (e.g., off-label drug prescribing)
- Long-range risks or risks to others (e.g., to children born of IVF). If these are not known, reveal the uncertainty.
- Subsequently learned information that has a bearing on a former patient's condition

How to Disclose

- Recognize that charisma and/or a referral from the patient's primary care physician may have the effect of overcoming patient concerns too readily and rendering a patient willing to accept any recommendation.
- In such cases, consider using an objective source to provide patient information about proposed treatment.
- If possible, give the patient time to reflect on the information before consenting.

IS THERE A PROFESSIONAL DUTY TO LEARN AND TO EDUCATE OTHER PRACTITIONERS?

A consistent theme that arose in the case study discussions at the Lasker Forum was the "duty to learn" (with the implication being that once learning takes place, it should be shared or taught). This topic deals with the problem that results when medical practice is altered but no evidence is collected on the impact of the change on patients or practice. Some physicians attempt new treatments and procedures and erroneously believe they are succeeding because they have plausible but undocumented explanations for why any failures were unrelated to the innovative aspect of treatment. It is only when data is collected on many cases and analyzed that errors become clear. Some physicians attempt innovations, fail, and never report their experiences, leaving open the possibility that other physicians will make the same mistake. Still other physicians succeed and do report their data but do so only selectively, leaving out some cases or information about problems, especially if disclosure might open the physician to criticism or liability. Other physicians are dissuaded from publishing for fear that they will be chastised (or worse) for having previously failed to classify a procedure as research and to seek IRB preapproval. Finally, some surgeons will not disclose or pass on their new skills because they want to retain what they consider to be professional secrets. Whatever the reason for refraining, failing to disseminate information on medical and surgical innovations deprives other professionals of valuable information that might prompt them to improve their patient care or jettison worthless or unsafe procedures. The end result is that patients suffer.

After discussing ways to remedy the problem, the Lasker Forum participants agreed that all innovating physicians should assume a duty to learn and to educate about the impact of their changes on patient care. Such a duty would require physicians to keep systematic records of innovative changes and outcomes on patients and, in the case of assisted reproductive technology, offspring. Technologies such as ART should also be subject to broader ranging data collection, for instance, on stored embryonic tissue samples. If a duty to learn exists, it follows that there is also a corresponding duty to disclose the outcome findings so that other physicians can be guided by the successes and failures of their colleagues. Otherwise, because there are so many ways that poor outcomes can be explained in medicine, physicians will continue to prescribe new therapies for longer than is justified. One Lasker Forum participant who has advocated a duty to learn and has been ignored in the past, cited high-dose chemotherapy with bone marrow transplant treatment for breast cancer in support of his view.

> These doctors believed so fervently that they knew how to produce the best results that they were willing to impose their beliefs on the patients. My group did one trial on bone marrow transplants for breast cancer that failed to show the benefit of this treatment. It took us eight years to enroll 800 women, during a time when 20,000 women were treated with bone marrow transplant outside of clinical trials. The difficulty here is that if the doctor believes the innovation is real, it may have nothing to do with the innovation. For instance, Dr. Oldwest in the assisted reproductive technology case may get better outcomes, but perhaps it's because he selects better couples and his outcomes have nothing to do with his techniques or his medium. Unless this is tested, we can't determine why his outcomes are good.

If formal research is not conducted, he went on, the least that innovating physicians can do is to collect outcome data on their patients and use it to inform themselves and other physicians.

A segment of the medical profession has always assumed these duties. Physicians have a history of publishing short anecdotal case reports of how they managed a particularly difficult or aberrant case or series of cases. As discussed in the Introduction, there is a tendency for case report findings to be adopted without the benefit of research validation. Yet, in the absence of research information, case reports are valuable (albeit erratic) sources of information because they provide insights that can improve the practice of medicine. Also, there are instances when groups of physicians voluntarily share outcome information about their innovations, such as is done online in the New England region (by the Northern New England Cardiovascular Disease Study Group via the website www.dartmouth.edu/~Ecardio/research/nnecdsg.htm). As with case study reporting, sharing within a study group or other form of consortium is voluntary and inconsistently done. If there is a duty to learn and educate about innovative medical technologies, outcomes reporting should somehow be broadened, regularized, and systemized by physicians who innovate outside of regulated research.

Agreeing that a duty to learn and educate exists does not mean that the issue is settled, however. There remain questions about what kinds of innovative changes would trigger a duty to collect and disseminate data. The duty exists most compellingly in cases of significant innovation accompanied by significant uncertainty about the innovation's impact. Also, whose duty is this precisely? Opinions on who has the responsibility seem to depend on the level of tolerance for outside intervention into professional practice, hence, suggestions range from physicians, clinics, and professional societies to states and the federal government. Finally, how can such a duty be imposed without undue burden? There is no consensus about whether data collection and dissemination should be considered an onerous part of the practice of medicine. One Lasker Forum participant suggested that, just as airline pilots do not consider redundant postflight routines to be a burden, neither should physicians who choose to innovate outside of a research environment consider recording, collecting, and disseminating data an extraordinary expectation. Both should be considered a part of regular responsible practice. On the other end of the burden perspective are physicians who fear that routine collection of outcome data on innovations will tend to transform all of medical innovation into research. Regardless of the disagreements over how it should be done, assessing outcomes in the field of innovative medicine is an unmet collective responsibility of the profession, and it deserves further consideration.

Final Thoughts on the Landscape of Innovation

Shortly before this book went to press, the *New York Times* reported on an operation performed on Vice President Dick Cheney (Altman 2005). The procedure involved the placement of stent-grafts to repair aneurysms in the arteries behind both knees. One day after the surgery, the vice president was reportedly doing well. However, surgeons and interventional radiologists were debating the wisdom of what had been done. The stent-grafts had not been approved by the FDA for use in knee vessels, and their use for this purpose was therefore considered off-label and innovative. No one knew, for instance, if these devices could withstand the constant knee motion to which they would be subjected. In addition, the intent initially was to operate on only one knee, but during the surgery the surgeons had decided to do both, which doubled the operative time to six hours and created unknown risks of complications. Presumably, if the operating surgeons had been allowed to speak to the press, they would have supported their work. Other surgeons who did speak to the *Times* reporter, however, expressed concern about both choices, to use the devices in the knees and to operate on both knees at once. The fact that these issues about an innovative surgery appeared in this article is evidence that they have risen in the public interest. It is also an indication, we think, of the timeliness of addressing the topic of how to deploy innovative medical technology.

The ethical challenge in this area is one with which one of us (DK) became familiar as commissioner of the Food and Drug Administration in the late 1970s. On the one hand, new technologies and new procedures offer the possibility of dramatic short-term benefit—even rescue—for the patient under treatment. On the other hand, premature introduction of those technologies or procedures presents real risks of iatrogenic illness; they may damage more than they cure. So the purpose of regulation, whether in the form of patient protection systems or of restraints on the approval of new drugs and devices, is to slow the deployment of technology until it has been thoroughly examined for risk. That effort can lead to lively arguments. FDA commissioners are often asked, as a challenge, whether the process of approving new drugs at the FDA might not slow the progress of innovation. The answer is, "of course." Regulation seeks to find a public policy position that balances the costs of premature introduction against the costs of forgone innovation. Those responsible for health policy constantly face a crossfire of charges: that they are not doing enough to protect patients and that they are doing harm to patients by forestalling innovation. This is an old dilemma in medicine, and it will be with us for some time.

This book and the Lasker Forum on Ethical Challenges in Biomedical Research and Practice on which the book is based are attempts to address this dilemma, in the process sketching the landscape of the current ethical and social issues associated with innovative medical technology. The medical literature, the lay press, and the forum discussions indicate that views on the topic of medical innovation range widely, from great optimism to extreme caution. Despite this disparity, there is agreement that innovative medical technology should be viewed in a social and ethical context. Some issues have been classified as valleys in the landscape, receiving little attention. For instance, access to new technology and social justice have received relatively less attention, perhaps because, as one forum participant put it, "we can't do anything about them in today's medical system, so why even discuss them?" Other issues rise up unavoidably, like peaks in the landscape, having more importance or being more amenable to resolution. These issues tend to receive the bulk of the attention. They include the main question, whether medical innovation should be deployed as research or as medical practice, and subsidiary questions like what oversight might be appropriate for unregulated technology, what disclosure duties exist when patients are first exposed to unproven medical technologies, and whether physicians have a duty to learn about the benefits and risks of their innovations and to pass this learning on to their colleagues.

On the overarching question of whether research or medical practice settings best serve medical innovation, the general assessment seems to be that not unless a particular new technology poses an unacceptable risk is deployment under a formal research protocol recommended. Although there were innovation-related problems in each of the four medical practice areas discussed here (off-label drug use, innovative surgery, assisted reproduction, and neuroimaging), those problems did not rise to a level that required the medical technologies to be researched before being offered as patient care. Nor is such an approach considered feasible. Instead, the focus should be on whether the process of medical innovation can be improved in less formal ways, namely, with nongovernmental oversight for some technologies and, for all technologies, better patient disclosure and better collection and publication of outcome data while innovating.

The first implication of these conclusions is that oversight, disclosure, and the duties to learn and educate are important considerations that should always be addressed when deploying new medical technologies. Oversight is important to prevent scientific enthusiasm from leading to uncritical acceptance and a limited view of the wider consequences of medical innovation. It is equally important to ensure that oversight does not unduly inhibit innovation. Using significant risk to identify the technologies that need oversight addresses this concern. Disclosure focuses on the patient, the ultimate beneficiary and sometimes the unfortunate victim of medical technology. Any attempt to address the ethical aspects of medical innovation needs to address the primary interest that must be given to patients' rights and must ensure that the imperatives of medical progress and social benefit do not trump these rights. The duties to learn and educate ensure that the information and the lessons, both good and bad, generated by an innovation are captured and disseminated. Learning and educating promote progress and can prevent the harm caused to patients when a lack of outside scrutiny perpetuates the use of an ineffective or unsafe medical technology.

The second implication of focusing on these three core concerns is that the lack of consensus in the medical profession regarding appropriate levels of oversight, patient consent, and information sharing must be tackled. There is a wide range of opinion about what standards are appropriate in these three areas, who should set the standards, and how each area should be managed. What constitutes appropriate technology oversight is a perennially debated topic among policy makers and society in general. There is no general agreement on which aspects of medical innovation should be left to the discretion of the profession (presumably the aspects that it knows and manages best) and which require extramural oversight. Accepting the primacy of patient autonomy has also led to ongoing debates about what constitutes an informed and free choice to accept or reject new medical treatment (the risks and benefits of which may be technical and opaque to both the practitioner and the patient). And, while there is general agreement that learning from and disseminating information about medical innovations are worthy goals, no agreement exists about how to accomplish them. The range of opinions on these topics indicates that further exploration of the landscape should focus on developing standards or best practices in these three areas.

The goal, after all, is for advances in medical technology to optimally serve the interests of science, medical practice, patients, and society. Success will depend first on understanding how medical innovations are being deployed and on identifying the issues that arise from that process. We have made an effort to contribute to these first steps, and we hope that this text will enrich continuing education on this topic, one that is so important to the role of medicine in society and to our collective future health.

Directives for
Human Experimentation:
Nuremberg Code

1. The voluntary consent of the human subject is absolutely essential. This means that the person involved should have legal capacity to give consent; should be so situated as to be able to exercise free power of choice, without the intervention of any element of force, fraud, deceit, duress, over-reaching, or other ulterior form of constraint or coercion; and should have sufficient knowledge and comprehension of the elements of the subject matter involved as to enable him to make an understanding and enlightened decision. This latter element requires that before the acceptance of an affirmative decision by the experimental subject there should be made known to him the nature, duration, and purpose of the experiment; the method and means by which it is to be conducted; all inconveniences and hazards reasonable to be expected; and the effects upon his health or person which may possibly come from his participation in the experiment.

2. The duty and responsibility for ascertaining the quality of the consent rests upon each individual who initiates, directs or engages in the experiment. It is a personal duty and responsibility which may not be delegated to another with impunity.

3. The experiment should be such as to yield fruitful results for the good of society, unprocurable by other methods or means of study, and not random and unnecessary in nature.

4. The experiment should be so designed and based on the results of animal experimentation and a knowledge of the natural history of the disease or other problem under study that the anticipated results will justify the performance of the experiment.

5. The experiment should be so conducted as to avoid all unnecessary physical and mental suffering and injury.

6. No experiment should be conducted where there is an a priori reason to believe that death or disabling injury will occur; except, perhaps, in those experiments where the experimental physicians also serve as subjects.

7. The degree of risk to be taken should never exceed that determined by the humanitarian importance of the problem to be solved by the experiment.

8. Proper preparations should be made and adequate facilities provided to protect the experimental subject against even remote possibilities of injury, disability, or death.

9. The experiment should be conducted only by scientifically qualified persons. The highest degree of skill and care should be required through all stages of the experiment of those who conduct or engage in the experiment.

10. During the course of the experiment the human subject should be at liberty to bring the experiment to an end if he has reached the physical or mental state where continuation of the experiment seems to him to be impossible.

11. During the course of the experiment the scientist in charge must be prepared to terminate the experiment at any stage if he has probable cause to believe, in the exercise of good faith, superior skill and careful judgment required of him, that a continuation of the experiment is likely to result in injury, disability, or death to the experimental subject.

SOURCE: National Institutes of Health, Office of Human Subjects Research, at http://ohsr.od.nih.gov/ guidelines/nuremberg.html. Reprinted from *Trials of War Criminals before the Nuremberg Military Tribunals under Control Council Law No. 10*, vol. 2, pp. 181–82. Washington, D.C.: U.S. Government Printing Office, 1949.

APPENDIX B

World Medical Association Declaration of Helsinki: Ethical Principles for Medical Research Involving Human Subjects

Adopted by the 18th WMA General Assembly, Helsinki, Finland, June 1964, and amended by the 29th WMA General Assembly, Tokyo, Japan, October 1975; 35th WMA General Assembly, Venice, Italy, October 1983; 41st WMA General Assembly, Hong Kong, September 1989; 48th WMA General Assembly, Somerset West, Republic of South Africa, October 1996; and the 52nd WMA General Assembly, Edinburgh, Scotland, October 2000.

Note of Clarification on Paragraph 29 added by the WMA General Assembly, Washington 2002.

Note of Clarification on Paragraph 30 added by the WMA General Assembly, Tokyo 2004.

A. INTRODUCTION

1. The World Medical Association has developed the Declaration of Helsinki as a statement of ethical principles to provide guidance to physicians and other participants in medical research involving human subjects. Medical research involving human subjects includes research on identifiable human material or identifiable data.

2. It is the duty of the physician to promote and safeguard the health of the people. The physician's knowledge and conscience are dedicated to the fulfillment of this duty.

3. The Declaration of Geneva of the World Medical Association binds the physician with the words, "The health of my patient will be my first considera-

tion," and the International Code of Medical Ethics declares that, "A physician shall act only in the patient's interest when providing medical care which might have the effect of weakening the physical and mental condition of the patient."

4. Medical progress is based on research which ultimately must rest in part on experimentation involving human subjects.

5. In medical research on human subjects, considerations related to the well-being of the human subject should take precedence over the interests of science and society.

6. The primary purpose of medical research involving human subjects is to improve prophylactic, diagnostic and therapeutic procedures and the understanding of the aetiology and pathogenesis of disease. Even the best proven prophylactic, diagnostic, and therapeutic methods must continuously be challenged through research for their effectiveness, efficiency, accessibility and quality.

7. In current medical practice and in medical research, most prophylactic, diagnostic and therapeutic procedures involve risks and burdens.

8. Medical research is subject to ethical standards that promote respect for all human beings and protect their health and rights. Some research populations are vulnerable and need special protection. The particular needs of the economically and medically disadvantaged must be recognized. Special attention is also required for those who cannot give or refuse consent for themselves, for those who may be subject to giving consent under duress, for those who will not benefit personally from the research and for those for whom the research is combined with care.

9. Research Investigators should be aware of the ethical, legal and regulatory requirements for research on human subjects in their own countries as well as applicable international requirements. No national ethical, legal or regulatory requirement should be allowed to reduce or eliminate any of the protections for human subjects set forth in this Declaration.

B. BASIC PRINCIPLES FOR ALL MEDICAL RESEARCH

10. It is the duty of the physician in medical research to protect the life, health, privacy, and dignity of the human subject.

11. Medical research involving human subjects must conform to generally accepted scientific principles, be based on a thorough knowledge of the scientific literature, other relevant sources of information, and on adequate laboratory and, where appropriate, animal experimentation.

12. Appropriate caution must be exercised in the conduct of research which may affect the environment, and the welfare of animals used for research must be respected.

13. The design and performance of each experimental procedure involving human subjects should be clearly formulated in an experimental protocol. This protocol should be submitted for consideration, comment, guidance, and, where appropriate, approval to a specially appointed ethical review committee, which must be independent of the investigator, the sponsor or any other kind of undue influence. This independent committee should be in conformity with the laws and regulations of the country in which the research experiment is performed. The committee has the right to monitor ongoing trials. The researcher has the obligation to provide monitoring information to the committee, especially any serious adverse events. The researcher should also submit to the committee, for review, information regarding funding, sponsors, institutional affiliations, other potential conflicts of interest and incentives for subjects.

14. The research protocol should always contain a statement of the ethical considerations involved and should indicate that there is compliance with the principles enunciated in this Declaration.

15. Medical research involving human subjects should be conducted only by scientifically qualified persons and under the supervision of a clinically competent medical person. The responsibility for the human subject must always rest with a medically qualified person and never rest on the subject of the research, even though the subject has given consent.

16. Every medical research project involving human subjects should be preceded by careful assessment of predictable risks and burdens in comparison with foreseeable benefits to the subject or to others. This does not preclude the participation of healthy volunteers in medical research. The design of all studies should be publicly available.

17. Physicians should abstain from engaging in research projects involving human subjects unless they are confident that the risks involved have been adequately assessed and can be satisfactorily managed. Physicians should cease any investigation if the risks are found to outweigh the potential benefits or if there is conclusive proof of positive and beneficial results.

18. Medical research involving human subjects should only be conducted if the importance of the objective outweighs the inherent risks and burdens to the subject. This is especially important when the human subjects are healthy volunteers.

19. Medical research is only justified if there is a reasonable likelihood that the populations in which the research is carried out stand to benefit from the results of the research.

20. The subjects must be volunteers and informed participants in the research project.

21. The right of research subjects to safeguard their integrity must always be respected. Every precaution should be taken to respect the privacy of the subject, the confidentiality of the patient's information and to minimize the impact of the study on the subject's physical and mental integrity and on the personality of the subject.

22. In any research on human beings, each potential subject must be adequately informed of the aims, methods, sources of funding, any possible conflicts of interest, institutional affiliations of the researcher, the anticipated benefits and potential risks of the study and the discomfort it may entail. The subject should be informed of the right to abstain from participation in the study or to withdraw consent to participate at any time without reprisal. After ensuring that the subject has understood the information, the physician should then obtain the subject's freely-given informed consent, preferably in writing. If the consent cannot be obtained in writing, the non-written consent must be formally documented and witnessed.

23. When obtaining informed consent for the research project the physician should be particularly cautious if the subject is in a dependent relationship with the physician or may consent under duress. In that case the informed consent should be obtained by a well-informed physician who is not engaged in the investigation and who is completely independent of this relationship.

24. For a research subject who is legally incompetent, physically or mentally incapable of giving consent or is a legally incompetent minor, the investigator must obtain informed consent from the legally authorized representative in accordance with applicable law. These groups should not be included in research unless the research is necessary to promote the health of the population represented and this research cannot instead be performed on legally competent persons.

25. When a subject deemed legally incompetent, such as a minor child, is able to give assent to decisions about participation in research, the investigator must obtain that assent in addition to the consent of the legally authorized representative.

26. Research on individuals from whom it is not possible to obtain consent, including proxy or advance consent, should be done only if the physical/mental condition that prevents obtaining informed consent is a necessary characteristic of the

research population. The specific reasons for involving research subjects with a condition that renders them unable to give informed consent should be stated in the experimental protocol for consideration and approval of the review committee. The protocol should state that consent to remain in the research should be obtained as soon as possible from the individual or a legally authorized surrogate.

27. Both authors and publishers have ethical obligations. In publication of the results of research, the investigators are obliged to preserve the accuracy of the results. Negative as well as positive results should be published or otherwise publicly available. Sources of funding, institutional affiliations and any possible conflicts of interest should be declared in the publication. Reports of experimentation not in accordance with the principles laid down in this Declaration should not be accepted for publication.

C. ADDITIONAL PRINCIPLES FOR MEDICAL RESEARCH COMBINED WITH MEDICAL CARE

28. The physician may combine medical research with medical care, only to the extent that the research is justified by its potential prophylactic, diagnostic or therapeutic value. When medical research is combined with medical care, additional standards apply to protect the patients who are research subjects.

29. The benefits, risks, burdens and effectiveness of a new method should be tested against those of the best current prophylactic, diagnostic, and therapeutic methods. This does not exclude the use of placebo, or no treatment, in studies where no proven prophylactic, diagnostic or therapeutic method exists. See footnote.

30. At the conclusion of the study, every patient entered into the study should be assured of access to the best proven prophylactic, diagnostic and therapeutic methods identified by the study. See footnote.

31. The physician should fully inform the patient which aspects of the care are related to the research. The refusal of a patient to participate in a study must never interfere with the patient-physician relationship.

32. In the treatment of a patient, where proven prophylactic, diagnostic and therapeutic methods do not exist or have been ineffective, the physician, with informed consent from the patient, must be free to use unproven or new prophylactic, diagnostic and therapeutic measures, if in the physician's judgment it offers hope of saving life, re-establishing health or alleviating suffering. Where possible, these measures should be made the object of research, designed to evaluate their safety and efficacy. In all cases, new information should be recorded

and, where appropriate, published. The other relevant guidelines of this Declaration should be followed.

Note: Note of clarification on paragraph 29 of the WMA Declaration of Helsinki

The WMA hereby reaffirms its position that extreme care must be taken in making use of a placebo-controlled trial and that in general this methodology should only be used in the absence of existing proven therapy. However, a placebo-controlled trial may be ethically acceptable, even if proven therapy is available, under the following circumstances:

- Where for compelling and scientifically sound methodological reasons its use is necessary to determine the efficacy or safety of a prophylactic, diagnostic or therapeutic method; or
- Where a prophylactic, diagnostic or therapeutic method is being investigated for a minor condition and the patients who receive placebo will not be subject to any additional risk of serious or irreversible harm.

All other provisions of the Declaration of Helsinki must be adhered to, especially the need for appropriate ethical and scientific review.

Note: Note of clarification on paragraph 30 of the WMA Declaration of Helsinki

The WMA hereby reaffirms its position that it is necessary during the study planning process to identify post-trial access by study participants to prophylactic, diagnostic and therapeutic procedures identified as beneficial in the study or access to other appropriate care. Post-trial access arrangements or other care must be described in the study protocol so the ethical review committee may consider such arrangements during its review.

The Declaration of Helsinki (Document 17.C) is an official policy document of the World Medical Association, the global representative body for physicians. It was first adopted in 1964 (Helsinki, Finland) and revised in 1975 (Tokyo, Japan), 1983 (Venice, Italy), 1989 (Hong Kong), 1996 (Somerset-West, South Africa) and 2000 (Edinburgh, Scotland). Note of clarification on Paragraph 29 added by the WMA General Assembly, Washington 2002.

SOURCE: World Medical Association, www.wma.net/e/policy/b3.htm, September 10, 2004.
NOTE: The Declaration of Helsinki is an official policy document of the World Medical Association (WMA), the global representative body for physicians.

Description of Department of Health and Human Services Regulations for the Protection of Human Subjects

At Title 45, Code of Federal Regulations, Part 46 (45 CFR Part 46), the U.S. Department of Health and Human Services has codified its regulations for the protection of human subjects. There are four subparts:

Subpart A (last revised June 18, 1991) is the Basic DHHS Policy for Protection of Human Research Subjects. Sixteen other federal departments and agencies are also formally bound to identical text by statute, regulation, or executive order.

Subpart B (last revised November 3, 1978) identifies Additional DHHS Protections Pertaining to Research, Development, and Related Activities Involving Fetuses, Pregnant Women, and Human in Vitro Fertilization. Subpart B is currently undergoing review in the department.

Subpart C (last revised November 16, 1978) identifies Additional DHHS Protections Pertaining to Biomedical and Behavioral Research Involving Prisoners as Subjects.

Subpart D (last revised March 8, 1983) identifies Additional DHHS Protections for Children Involved as Subjects in Research.

The local Institutional Review Board (IRB) at the research site is the cornerstone of this system of protection of human subjects. No human subjects research may be initiated, and no ongoing research may continue, in the absence of IRB approval. HHS cannot provide funds for, or conduct, human subjects research unless one or more IRB's approves the protocol for such studies.

An IRB is established at the local level and, by regulation, has a minimum of five people, including at least one scientist, one nonscientist, and one person not otherwise affiliated with that institution.

IRB review is a prospective as well as continuing review of research by a group of individuals. In reviewing research, IRB's must be knowledgeable about the research site; the resources of the institution; the capabilities and reputations of the investigators and staff; and the prevailing values and ethics of the community and, most important, the likely subject population.

In order to approve research, the IRB must determine that all of the following requirements are satisfied:

1. Risks to human subjects are minimized.
2. Risks to human subjects are reasonable in relation to anticipated benefits, if any, to human subjects, and the importance of the knowledge that may reasonably be expected to result.
3. Selection of human subjects is equitable.
4. Informed consent will be sought from each prospective human subject or the human subject's legally authorized representative, in accordance with, and to the extent required by 45 CFR Part 46.
5. Informed consent will be appropriately documented in accordance with and to the extent required by 45 CFR Part 46.
6. When appropriate, the research plan makes adequate provision for monitoring the data collected to ensure the safety of human subjects.
7. When appropriate, there are adequate, provisions to protect the privacy of human subjects and to maintain the confidentiality of data.

In addition, when some or all of the human subjects are likely to be vulnerable to coercion or undue influence, additional safeguards have been included in the study to protect the rights and welfare of these human subjects.

Once research is underway, the IRB must conduct continuing review of the research, at intervals appropriate to the degree of risk—in any event, at least once per year.

Continuing review is substantive and meaningful. In approving the continuation of ongoing research, an IRB attests to its satisfaction that the research continues to be conducted in accord with all relevant provisions of the regulations.

IRB's also oversee the informed consent process. The regulations specify eight required elements of informed consent:

1. A statement that the study involves research, an explanation of the purposes of the research and the expected duration of the subject's participation, a description of the procedures to be followed, and identification of any procedures which are experimental.

2. A description of any reasonably foreseeable risks or discomforts to the subject.

3. A description of any benefits to the subject or to others which may reasonably be expected from the research.

4. A disclosure of appropriate alternative procedures or courses of treatment, if any, that might be advantageous to the subject.

5. A statement describing the extent, if any, to which confidentiality of records identifying the subject will be maintained.

6. For research involving more than minimal risk, an explanation as to whether any compensation and an explanation as to whether any medical treatments are available if injury occurs and, if so, what they, consist of, or where further information may be obtained.

7. An explanation of whom to contact for answers to pertinent questions about the research and research subjects' rights, and whom to contact in the event of a research-related injury to the subject.

8. A statement that participation is voluntary, refusal to participate will involve no penalty or loss of benefits to which the subject is otherwise entitled and the subject may discontinue participation at any time without penalty or loss of benefits to which the subject is otherwise entitled.

SOURCE: Director, Office for Protection from Research Risks, Testimony on Protection of Human Research Subjects, March 12, 1996. Available from www.hhs.gov/asl/testify/t960312a.html.

Participants in Lasker Forum on Ethical Challenges in Biomedical Research and Practice

PLANNING COMMITTEE

Paul Berg, Ph.D.
Nobel Laureate, Cahill Professor of Cancer Research, Emeritus
Stanford University Medical School

R. Alta Charo, J.D.
Professor of Law and Medical Ethics
University of Wisconsin Law School and Medical School

James F. Childress, Ph.D.
Professor of Ethics
University of Virginia

Ruth R. Faden, Ph.D., M.P.H.
Professor and Executive Director
The Phoebe R. Berman Bioethics Institute
Johns Hopkins University Bloomberg School of Public Health

Mark Frankel, Ph.D.
Director, Program on Scientific Freedom, Responsibility, and Law
American Association for the Advancement of Science

Vanessa Gamble, M.D., Ph.D.
Director, National Center for Bioethics in Research and Health Care
Tuskegee University

Henry T. Greely, J.D.
Professor of Law
Stanford University

U.S. Senator Mark Hatfield
Portland, Oregon

Rudolf Jaenisch, M.D.
Whitehead Institute for Biomedical Research

Donald Kennedy, Ph.D. (co-chair)
President Emeritus, Stanford University
Editor-in-Chief, *Science*

Mary-Claire King, Ph.D.
Professor of Medicine and Genetics
University of Washington School of Medicine

Bernard Lo, M.D.
Professor of Medicine
University of California, San Francisco

Jessica Mathews, Ph.D.
President, Carnegie Endowment for International Peace

Thomas H. Murray, Ph.D.
President, The Hastings Center

Harold T. Shapiro, Ph.D. (co-chair)
President Emeritus, Princeton University
Former Chair, National Bioethics Advisory Commission

LeRoy B. Walters, Ph.D.
Joseph P. Kennedy Sr. Professor of Christian Ethics
Kennedy Institute of Ethics

Rick Weiss
The Washington Post

For the Mary Woodard Lasker Charitable Trust and Foundation

Neen Hunt, Ed.D., President
Martin Krasney, Coordinator
Margaret L. Eaton, Pharm.D., J.D., Lasker Forum researcher and case writer

ATTENDEES

Dr. Grover C. Bagby, Oregon Health and Sciences University
Dr. Patricia Baird, University of British Columbia
Mr. Robert Bazell, NBC News
Dr. Paul Berg, Stanford University Medical Center
Dr. Elizabeth Blackburn, University of California, San Francisco
Ms. Susan Brink, *U.S. News and World Report*
Mr. W. Michael Brown, Lasker Foundation
Dr. John H. Campbell, University of California, Los Angeles
Dr. Christine Cassel, Oregon Health and Sciences University
Dr. Lynn Cates, Veterans Health Administration
Dr. R. Alta Charo, University of Wisconsin Law School and Medical School
Dr. James F. Childress, University of Virginia Center for Biomedical Ethics
Dr. Bette Jane Crigger, Veterans Health Administration
Ms. Barbara J. Culliton, The Institute for Genomic Research
Dr. Rebecca Susan Dresser, Washington University School of Law
Dr. Margaret L. Eaton, Stanford University
Dr. Ruth Faden, Johns Hopkins University Bloomberg School of Public Health
Rabbi David Feldman, The Jewish Institute of Bioethics
Mr. James W. Fordyce, Lasker Foundation
Mr. Stephen Foster, The Overbrook Foundation
Dr. Mark Frankel, American Association for the Advancement of Science
Ms. Susan Grandis Goldstein, *Religion and News Weekly*
Mr. Henry T. Greely, Stanford University

Dr. Kathy Hudson, Johns Hopkins University Bioethics Institute

Mr. James E. Hughes, Lasker Foundation

Dr. Neen Hunt, Lasker Trust and Foundation

Mr. Peter Barton Hutt, Covington and Burling

Dr. Judy Illes, Stanford University

Dr. Jeffrey Kahn, University of Minnesota

Dr. Nancy Kass, Johns Hopkins University Bloomberg School of Public Health

Dr. Donald Kennedy, Stanford University

Dr. Patricia A. King, Georgetown University Law Center

Dr. Michael Klag, Johns Hopkins University School of Medicine

Ms. Lori P. Knowles, The Hastings Center

Dr. Greg Koski, Harvard Medical School

Mr. Martin Krasney

Dr. Jennifer Kulynych, Ropes and Gray

Dr. David Lepay, Food and Drug Administration

Dr. Bernard Lo, University of California, San Francisco

Dr. Peter Lurie, Public Citizen's Health Research Group

Dr. David Magnus, University of Pennsylvania

Dr. Anna Mastroianni, University of Washington School of Law

Dr. Richard Merrill, University of Virginia Law School

Dr. Jon F. Merz, University of Pennsylvania

Dr. Jonathan D. Moreno, University of Virginia

Dr. Thomas H. Murray, The Hastings Center

Dr. Craig Nichols, Oregon Health and Science University

Dr. Philip Noguchi, Food and Drug Administration

Judge John T. Noonan, U.S. Court of Appeals, Ninth Circuit

Dr. Sherwin B. Nuland, Yale University School of Medicine

Dr. Pilar N. Ossorio, University of Wisconsin Law School

Dr. Patrick Reilly, Association of Clinical Research Professionals

Dr. John A. Robertson, University of Texas School of Law

Dr. Karen J. Rothenberg, University of Maryland School of Law

Dr. William M. Sage, Columbia School of Law

Dr. Richard Schilsky, University of Chicago Hospitals and Health System

Ms. Noel Schwerin, Backbone Media

Dr. Harold T. Shapiro, Princeton University

Dr. Lee M. Silver, Princeton University

Dr. Gregory B. Stock, University of California, Los Angeles

Mr. William C. Stubing, The Greenwall Foundation

Dr. Jeremy Sugarman, Duke University
Mrs. Leslie Tucker, The Pew Charitable Trusts
Dr. LeRoy Walters, Georgetown University
Dr. Simon Whitney, Baylor College of Medicine
Dr. Keith Yamamoto, University of California, San Francisco
Dr. Paul Yock, Stanford University

Notes

PREFACE

1. One of the objectives of the Albert and Mary Lasker Foundation is to enlarge public awareness, appreciation, and understanding of promising achievements in medical science in order to increase public support for research. The foundation believes that scientific investigation and knowledge of basic human biology and disease processes are the most reliable and efficient means by which to achieve prolongation of life and reduction of human suffering. The centerpiece event of the foundation is an annual awards program that recognizes transforming achievements in basic and clinical research and significant public service on behalf of medical science. See www.laskerfoundation.org.

2. Harold Shapiro is professor of economics and public policy and president emeritus of Princeton University and the former chair of the National Bioethics Advisory Commission, which advised President Bill Clinton on biomedical ethical matters.

3. A major issue inherent in the ethical nature of this gray area is where the boundaries lie between research and medical practice. This question was addressed in a systematic way in the 1970s during the preparation of the Belmont Report but, although discussed periodically in the medical literature, has not been dealt with in a comprehensive manner since. The Lasker Forum principals believed that the medical innovation climate had become so advanced and the related issues so much broader that a new look at the question was warranted. For a further discussion of the Belmont Report's work on this issue, see Chapter 1.

INTRODUCTION: THE NEED TO ASK QUESTIONS
ABOUT INNOVATION

The quotation from Sophocles is part of the "Ode to Man" chorus in *Antigone* and is taken from *The Three Theban Plays*, translated by Robert Fagles (New York: Penguin Books USA, 2000).

1. The primary ethical duties of physicians regarding the patients whom they recruit for human research have been derived from many research ethics codes and basically fall into the following categories: (1) to avoid exploiting vulnerable patients, (2) to minimize harm as much as possible and ensure that any risk of harm is not greater than the sum of the benefit to the subject and the importance of the knowledge to be gained, (3) to allow

patients to make fully informed and uncoerced autonomous decisions to participate as human subjects, (4) to respect subjects by ensuring medical privacy, allowing them to withdraw from the research, and monitoring their well-being, and (5) to competently conduct a scientifically valid study. See Emanuel, Wendler, and Grady 2000.

2. Moore 1988, 2000.

3. The combination of these study methods is described as prospective, randomized, placebo controlled, and double blind. Often called the gold standard for clinical medical research, this type of study is most often required by the FDA to support applications for approval of regulated medical products. Studies can also prospectively test the experimental treatment against another type of control, such as an alternative treatment. Other types of study control, such as comparisons with past treatments (historic controls), are considered statistically and medically weaker.

4. From this point on, this account of the diffusion of medical technology is roughly based on a thoughtful article, McKinlay 1981. Although written about twenty-five years ago, the progression of innovation described in the article remains accurate in many respects.

5. The parties eventually settled for a lower, undisclosed amount.

6. An institutional review board (IRB) is a committee whose purpose is to review and monitor biomedical research involving human subjects conducted in a particular institution. IRBs are generally composed of some combination of physicians, scientists, administrators, and community representatives. An IRB has the authority to approve, require modifications to, or disapprove a research proposal and to order a study terminated once under way, for various reasons. The fundamental purpose of an IRB review is to ensure that human subjects are given the opportunity to provide informed consent, that the risks to subjects are minimized, and that the rights and welfare of human subjects are optimally protected.

7. Prefrontal lobotomy, which was first used at the end of the 1800s and which changed over time, involved the use of surgical instruments to sever the prefrontal cortex from the rest of the brain. The intended outcome, which was variably achieved, was the pacification of highly agitated psychiatric patients. Antonio Moniz, of the University of Lisbon Medical School, was credited with generating the initial popularity of the procedure, and for his work he won the Nobel Prize in 1949.

8. Cingulotomy uses magnetic resonance imaging to stereotactically guide probes into the white matter of the cingulate gyrus of the brain. Heat is then generated from the tips of the probe to burn small areas of targeted brain tissue.

9. Typically, demonstrating safety and efficacy vis-à-vis placebo is all that is necessary for FDA approval of a drug, biologic, or medical device.

10. Coronary artery disease is caused by the accumulation of fat and cholesterol on the inside of coronary arteries. This accumulation leads to the formation of deposits called plaque, which grow so that they narrow and block the arteries that feed blood and oxygen to the heart. Coronary artery disease is one of the most common causes of premature death in North America.

11. Nitroglycerin was used for more than 100 years before researchers discovered that the drug's vasodilation action was caused by its release of nitric oxide. For their discovery of nitric oxide as a signaling molecule in the cardiovascular system, three U.S. researchers

won the 1998 Nobel Prize. Their discovery prompted a remarkable amount of pharmaco-logic research on the implications and uses of nitric oxide in hypertension (which has led to the drug BiDil), shock, pulmonary disorders, cancers, impotency (which led to the drug Viagra), and for diagnosing inflammatory disorders.

12. This initial history of coronary artery surgery draws from McKinlay 1981. The in-formation about more recent treatments for coronary artery disease is primarily from Med-line Plus (http://medlineplus.gov/).

13. CABG is a form of open heart surgery in which a detour or "bypass" is created around the blocked part of a coronary artery to restore the blood supply to the heart muscle. The bypass is created using pieces of veins or arteries from other parts of the patient's body.

14. The designation "percutaneous" is because the physician performing the proce-dure inserts all catheters, surgical tools, and substances through small cuts in the skin and then in a blood vessel. The catheters through which tools reach the heart are usually threaded through a cut in the groin, into the femoral artery, and then to the heart vessels. PTCA restores blood supply and oxygen to the heart by opening blocked or narrowed coro-nary blood vessels using small balloons. Other percutaneous procedures used to treat coro-nary artery disease are: coronary atherectomy (coronary vessel plaque tissue is shaved off), ablative laser-assisted angioplasty (laser probes remove plaque from vessel wall, then an-gioplasty is performed), catheter-based thrombolysis and mechanical thrombectomy (using catheter-delivered drugs or surgical tools to dissolve or remove blood clots in the coronary vessel), coronary stenting (insertion of a tube to keep the coronary vessel open [discussed further in the text]), coronary radiation implant or coronary brachytherapy (delivery of beta or gamma radiation into the coronary arteries; currently approved for patients who have failed with other stent-related procedures and is being studied at some centers as first-line treatment).

15. All of these technologies are regulated to some degree, ranging from slight to heavy.

16. The death in 1999 of 18-year-old Jesse Gelsinger in a University of Pennsylvania experiment in which the research protocol was not followed led to the government-enforced closure of the university's gene therapy research program, internal and congres-sional investigations, and the resignation of the director of the gene therapy program. This death also led to widespread debate about the adequacy of protections for human research subjects, the rapidity with which innovative physicians take new medical technologies from the laboratory bench to the bedside, and the influences of corporate funding on re-searchers' decision making. It also led to the fear that support for this promising new field of medicine would decline significantly. (See Marshall 2000.)

CHAPTER I. DISTINGUISHING INNOVATIVE
MEDICAL PRACTICE FROM RESEARCH

1. Among the inciting events were the infamous Tuskegee syphilis experiment and the 1966 revelations by Harvard University's Henry Beecher, published in the *New England Journal of Medicine*, of other ethically problematic human studies (Beecher 1966a, 1966b).

2. To Levine's list we add reproductive technologies, functional neural imaging, so-called natural or alternative remedies, and nutritional supplements.

3. Because of fears about medical risk, liability, and an inability to obtain parental consent for sufficient subjects, it was common for pharmaceutical companies to conduct research only in adults. This led to the situation in which most pediatric medical products were used without the benefit of research in children. In 2003, Congress passed the Pediatric Research Equity Act, a law that required pharmaceutical companies to conduct research in children if a new prescription drug or biologic substance is intended to treat a condition that affects both adults and children. Legal loopholes and the fact that it expires in 2007 have generated concerns that the law will not stimulate as much pediatric research as is needed. Significantly, the law does not apply to prescription drugs already on the market. As a result, use of many drugs, biologic substances, and devices in children will continue without first having been subjected to research.

4. The most prominent of these deaths was that of Jesse Gelsinger, described in Introduction note 16.

CHAPTER 2. THE MODERN HISTORY OF HUMAN RESEARCH ETHICS

1. In 2001, multiple project assurance was replaced by Federalwide Assurance (FWA).

CHAPTER 3. INNOVATION IN THE OFF-LABEL USE OF DRUGS

1. According to the Food and Drug Administration Modernization Act (FDAMA) of 1997, section 401, drug manufacturers can release qualified, objective, and balanced scientific information (mainly from unabridged peer-reviewed journal articles) about off-label uses of their drugs so long as they also provide data and/or conduct studies to support the submission of supplemental FDA applications to seek approval for those off-label uses. Exceptions include cases in which it would be "economically prohibitive" to make the FDA submissions or when the off-label use is so well accepted that it would be unethical to conduct the studies, because they would deprive the control subjects of the accepted therapy. The FDA has the authority to issue warning letters (but not fines), seek injunctions, or bring criminal charges against companies that violate the restrictions on off-label promotion. In 1994, the FDAMA and the regulatory restrictions on off-label promotion were challenged as an unconstitutional restriction on commercial free speech in *Washington Legal Foundation v. Jane Henney*. After years of appeals and rulings, the litigation was concluded without having settled a main question: whether the FDA would violate the manufacturer's First Amendment rights by prohibiting or penalizing off-label promotion outside of FDAMA's "safe harbor" provisions.

2. According to the FDA, 1 to 2 percent of new drugs are recalled from the market because of an unacceptable adverse reaction rate when used for an *approved* purpose. We know of no reliable data on adverse drug reaction rates for off-label uses.

CHAPTER 5. INNOVATION IN ASSISTED REPRODUCTION

1. IVF involves administering fertility drugs to a woman, surgically collecting the eggs she produces as a result, and placing the eggs with sperm from the male partner in a cul-

ture dish. If fertilization occurs, healthy-appearing embryos are implanted (via a surgical tube called a laparoscope) into the uterus of the woman. Sometimes a surrogate woman is sought to gestate the fetus. Embryos that are not implanted are frozen and stored in the lab. The facts of IVF—that any woman and any man can donate the gametes for IVF, that a different woman can gestate the fetus, and that some people donate their leftover embryos to others—have generated a host of legal and ethical disputes about parental rights and responsibilities.

2. In GIFT, sperm and eggs are placed directly into the woman's fallopian tube to foster fertilization.

3. In ZIFT, the fertilized egg is transferred back into the woman at the two-cell stage instead of the four- or eight-cell stage as with conventional IVF.

4. ICSI involves injecting sperm directly into the human egg to create the embryo.

5. HIPAA is the Health Insurance Portability and Accountability Act, which went into effect in April 2003 and governs the privacy and security of health-related information.

CHAPTER 6. INNOVATION IN NEUROIMAGING

1. Functional magnetic resonance imaging employs powerful magnetic fields noninvasively to monitor the rate of blood flow to the various parts of the brain. Because increased blood flow correlates with brain activity, the images produced with fMRI reveal which parts of the brain are active at the time. The technology has been used since the mid-1990s to understand the neurobiological basis for our behavior, for instance, by observing the regions of the brain that are responsible for learning, memory, and emotion. The combination of fMRI and more conventional MRI studies can provide simultaneous information on structure and function of the brain. Enough research has already been done with both forms of imaging to produce structural and functional brain images that are considered characteristic standards for many types of mental illness.

CHAPTER 7. QUESTIONS, ISSUES, AND RECOMMENDATIONS
GOING FORWARD

1. Balloon angioplasty is a surgical procedure in which a small balloon is inserted and inflated to open narrowed or blocked blood vessels of the heart (coronary arteries). A coronary stent is a semiflexible tube left in place to hold open the previously clogged artery. For further information about stent development, see the Introduction.

2. In the United Kingdom, IVF physicians are legally obliged to report ART results to a national registry. In the United States, any reporting is voluntary. See www.asrm.org for information about ASRM's ART registry.

3. According to the FDA, citing the *Code of Federal Regulations,* the terms *research* and *clinical investigation* mean "any experiment that involves a test article and one or more human subjects, and that either must meet the requirements for prior submission to the Food and Drug Administration under section 505(i), 507(d), or 520(g) of the act, or need not meet the requirements for prior submission to the Food and Drug Administration under these sections of the act, but the results of which are intended to be later submitted

to, or held for inspection by, the Food and Drug Administration as part of an application for a research or marketing permit" (21 CFR 56). The DHHS definition is broader and inclusive of the FDA definition. It is taken from the so-called Common Rule, which defines research as "a systematic investigation, including research development, testing, and evaluation, designed to develop or contribute to generalizable knowledge. Activities which meet this definition constitute research for purposes of this policy, whether or not they are conducted or supported under a program which is considered research for other purposes. For example, some demonstration and service programs may include research activities. A systematic investigation that is not designed to be generalizable is not 'research.' A quality assurance audit may be very systematic but is not designed to be generalizable; it is therefore not research." (See 45 CFR 46, subpart A.)

4. The committee membership includes staff physicians and representatives from biomedical engineering, health policy, patient care services, research, finance, clinical labs, critical care, ethics, legal affairs, and the Decision Support Unit. Members from two related entities also serve on the committee: the Center for Integration of Medicine and Innovative Technology, a nonprofit consortium that brings together scientists, engineers, and clinicians to improve patient care by catalyzing development of innovative technology; and the hospital's Institute for Technology. The committee develops and uses state-of-the-art methodologies for technology assessment and uses health outcomes research to guide the development, evaluation, and utilization of technologies that can improve the quality and cost-effectiveness of medical care. Together, committee members engage in a process of assessing the clinical effects of innovative medical technologies (safety, efficacy, degree of improvement over existing technology, need, regulatory requirements, and the social, ethical, and legal impacts). In addition, the committee addresses administrative questions such as how much the technology will cost, how it will affect the use of medical personnel, whether it will be cost effective, what the reimbursement opportunities are, whether its use fits into the strategic plan of the hospital, and what the risk management and legal liability issues and impacts are. With this information and using a process-improvement methodology, the committee decides whether to adopt the technology and, if so, whether it can be introduced as medical practice or offered only under a research protocol. The committee then monitors the use of the technology to determine the validity of the original information and assumptions about the technology and whether any revisions need to be made to improve the use of the technology. The authors thank the chair of the committee, Dr. Harold J. DeMonaco, for this information.

5. A paper on the history of continuous hemodialysis contains some interesting insights into the process of medical innovation. The author describes the mistake that led to the idea behind continuous dialysis technology (inserting a dialysis catheter into a patient's femoral artery instead of a vein), the deaths that resulted from unanticipated problems in early patients, and the various technical improvements that were attempted to maximize effectiveness (changing the diameter of catheters, using shorter tubes, designing special stopcocks, changing the composition and configuration of dialysis filters, changing pressures at the filter outlet, varying the placement of the fluid inlets and outlets on the filters, and many other small and complicated equipment details and physiology factors). The vagaries of this process led the author to state that "new ideas and techniques in medicine

rarely occur in a straightforward manner; they often originate from indistinct concepts or even incorrect assumptions, or they happen simply by accident. However, the pathway from noticing an event and pondering on an indistinct situation to the genesis of a useful and effective procedure depends on the fantasy and creativity of personalities and the firmness with which they promote the generative process. Once the potential of the idea becomes evident, its further development accelerates like a river that is progressively fed by many varied sources. The remarkable genesis of the continuous renal replacement techniques is an instructive example of this evolution" (Burchardi 1998, p. S120).

6. For more on AHRQ, see www.ahrqtap@ahrq.gov and www.ahcpr.gov/clinic/epc/.

7. Spina bifida falls within a class of neural tube defects in which the central nervous system (brain and spinal cord) does not form properly in the early stages of pregnancy. Each year in the United States, about 2,500 children are born with this medically complex but nonlethal defect, which is associated with full or partial paralysis, other neurological complications, hydrocephalus, difficulties with bladder and bowel control, learning disabilities, depression, and social and sexual issues.

8. In this study, the researchers employed a "nondirective counseling" consent process in accordance with the voluntary ethics guidelines developed by the International Fetal Medicine and Surgery Society.

9. While the surgery was shown to lessen the need for postnatal shunts to control hydrocephalus, the surgeon authors concluded that "it remains to be determined whether this benefit outweighs the potential risks of intrauterine surgery."

10. At the time of the Lasker Forum, Vanderbilt surgeons had performed about 200 of these surgeries and were busy working on techniques, including the use of robotics, to improve their success rates.

11. Another Lasker Forum participant, a representative of the news media, deplored this increasingly common phenomenon of patients rushing to seek treatment by saying, "Sometimes I really question my career. Information about medical advances is great news. But a lot of what we have done is feed expectations for perfect outcomes. Lost in this is the role of fate or God or chance. People now expect too much. Too few times do these news stories include the wide variation in perspective that exists."

References

Adamson, D. 2002. Regulation of assisted reproductive technologies in the United States. *Fertility and Sterility* 78 (November): 932–42.

Aetna Insurance. 2005. Stereotactic cingulotomy. *Aetna Clinical Bulletin*, August 2. Available from www.aetna.com/cpb/data/CPBA0288.html.

Altman, L.K. 2005. Vice president has surgery for aneurysm in each knee. *New York Times*, September 25, p. 14.

American Society of Reproductive Medicine. 1996. Fact sheet: Risks of in vitro fertilization. Available from www.asrm.org/Patients/FactSheets/RisksIVF-Fact.pdf.

Andrews, L.B. 1999. *Clone Age: Adventures in the New World of Reproductive Technology.* New York: Henry Holt.

Angell, M. 1997. The ethics of clinical research in the third world. *New England Journal of Medicine* 337:847–49.

Battling a Brain Tumor. 2000. *48 Hours*, CBS News, September 6. Available from www.cbsnews.com/stories/2000/09/01/48hours/main229989.shtml.

Beck, J.M., and Azari, E.D. 1997. FDA, off-label use and informed consent, debunking myths and misconceptions. *Food and Drug Law Journal* 53:71–104.

Beecher, H.K. 1966a. Consent in clinical experimentation: Myth and reality. *Journal of the American Medical Association* 195:34–35.

Beecher, H.K. 1966b. Ethics and clinical research. *New England Journal of Medicine* 274:1354–60.

Beecher, H.K. 1970. *Research and the Individual: Human Studies.* Boston: Little, Brown.

Belmont Report. 1979. Available from National Institutes of Health, Office of Human Subjects Research, at http://ohsr.od.nih.gov/guidelines/belmont.html.

Blank, R.H. 1997. Assisted reproduction and reproductive rights: The case of in vitro fertilization. *Politics and the Life Sciences* 16 (September): 279–88.

Blum, R.S. 2002. Legal considerations in off-label medication prescribing. *Archives of Internal Medicine* 162:1777–79.

Bonchek, L.I., and Ullyot, D.J. 1998. Minimally invasive coronary bypass: A dissenting opinion. *Circulation* 98:495–97.

Borst, C., and Grundeman, P.F. 1999. Minimally invasive coronary artery bypass grafting: An experimental perspective. *Circulation* 99:1400–1403.

Brorsson, B., Bernstein, S.J., and Herlitz, J. 1999. Four-year follow-up of patients with chronic stable angina referred for CABG, PTCA or medical treatment: Mortality, symptoms and well-being. *Annual Meeting of the International Society of Technology Assessment in Health Care* 15:63.

Brosgart, C.L., et al. 1996. Off-label drug use in human immunodeficiency virus disease. *Journal of Acquired Immune Deficiency Syndromes and Human Retrovirology* 12:56–62.

Brower, V. 2003. The ethics of innovation. *EMBO Reports* 4:338–40.

Bruner, J., Richards, W.O., Tulipan, N.B., et al. 1999. Endoscopic coverage of fetal myelomeningocele in utero. *American Journal of Obstetrics and Gynecology* 180:153–58.

Bunch, W.H., and Dvonch, V.M. 2000. Moral decisions regarding innovation. *Clinical Orthopaedics and Related Research* 378 (September): 44–49.

Bunker, J.P., Hinkley, D., and McDermott, W.V. 1978. Surgical innovation and its evaluation. *Science* 200:937–41.

Burchardi, H. 1998. History and development of continuous renal replacement techniques. *Kidney International—Critical Care Nephrology,* 53 suppl. 66:S120–24.

Canli, T., and Amin, Z. 2002. Neuroimaging of emotion and personality: Scientific evidence and ethical considerations. *Brain and Cognition* 50 (December): 414–31.

Centers for Disease Control and Prevention. 2003. Assisted Reproductive Technology Success Rates. Available from http://www.cdc.gov/ART/ARTReports.ntm#2003.

Charo, R.A. 2002. Children by choice: Reproductive technologies and the boundaries of personal autonomy. *Nature Cell Biology,* suppl., s23–s28.

Code of Federal Regulations, Protection of Human Subjects, Basic HHS Policy for Protection of Human Research Subjects, Title 45, Part 46, Subpart A.

Cohen, J. 1999. Behind the headlines of endostatin's ups and downs. *Science* 283:1250–51.

Colapinto, J. 2005. Bloodsuckers. *New Yorker,* July 25, p. 77.

Cooley, D., and Frazier, O.H. 2000. The past fifty years of cardiovascular surgery. *Circulation* 102 suppl. (November): IV-87–IV-93.

Cosgrove, G.R., and Rauch, S.L. 2003. Stereotactic cingulotomy. *Neurosurgery Clinics of North America* 14:225–35.

Desperately Fighting Cancer. 2002. *60 Minutes,* CBS News, April 4. Available at www.cbsnews.com/stories/2002/04/04/60minutes/main505402.shtml.

Dosseter, J.B. 1990. Innovative treatment versus clinical research: An ethics issue in transplantation. *Transplantation Proceedings* 22:966–68.

Eaton, M.L., Green, B., Church, T., and Niewoehner, D. 1980. Efficacy of theophylline in non-asthmatic obstructive airway disease. *Annals of Internal Medicine* 92:758–61.

Emanuel, E.J., Wendler, D., and Grady, C. 2000. What makes clinical research ethical? *Journal of the American Medical Association* 283:2701–11.

Farquhar, C., et al. 2005. High dose chemotherapy and autologous bone marrow or stem cell transplantation versus conventional chemotherapy for women with metastatic breast cancer. *Cochrane Database Systematic Reviews* 20(3):CD003142.

Federman, D.D., Hanna, K.E., and Rodriguez, L.L., eds. 2002. Responsible research: A systems approach to protecting research participants. Committee on Assessing the System for Protecting Human Research Participants, Institute of Medicine. Washington, D.C.: National Academy Press.

Flannery, E.J. 1986. Should it be easier or harder to use unapproved drugs and devices? *Hastings Center Report* 16:17–23.

Frederickson, D.S. 1968. The field trial: Some thoughts on the indispensable ordeal. *Bulletin of the New York Academy of Medicine* 44:985–93.

Frost, N. 1998. Ethical dilemmas in medical innovation and research: distinguishing experimentation from practice. *Seminars in Perinatology* 22:223–32.

Gallant, D. 1979. Response to commission duties as detailed in Public Law 93-348, sec. 202(a)(1)(B)(1). In National Commission for the Protection of Human Subjects of Biomedical and Behavioral Research, Boundaries between Research and Practice, Belmont Report, Appendix Volume II, DHEW Publication No. (OS) 78-0014.

Gawande, A. 2002. *Complications: A Surgeon's Notes on an Imperfect Science.* New York: Henry Holt, pp. 15–16.

Gawande, A. 2003. Desperate measures: Francis Moore remade modern surgery. But he couldn't live with the consequences. *New Yorker,* May 5.

Gindro, S., and Mordini, E. 1998. Ethical, legal and social issues in brain research. *Current Opinion in Psychiatry* 11 (September): 575–80.

Goldiamond, I. 1979. On the usefulness of intent for distinguishing between research and practice, and its replacement by social contingency: Implications for standard and innovative procedures, coercion and informed consent, and fiduciary and contractual relations. Page 14-4 in National Commission for the Protection of Human Subjects of Biomedical and Behavioral Research, Boundaries between Research and Practice, Belmont Report, Appendix Volume II, DHEW Publication No. (OS) 78-0014.

Greely, H.T. 2002. Neuroethics and ELSI: Some comparisons and considerations. Conference Proceedings, Neuroethics: Mapping the Field. Dana Foundation, San Francisco, May.

Groopman, J. 2003. The Reeve effect. *New Yorker,* November 10.

Heames, R.M., et al. 2002. Off-pump coronary artery surgery. *Anaesthesia* 57 (July): 676–85.

Illes, J., et al. 2003. From neuroimaging to neuroethics, *Nature Neuroscience* 6:250.

Johannes, L. 2004. A screening test for high-risk mothers. *Wall Street Journal,* November 23, p. D1.

Johnson, M.H. 2002. The art of regulation and the regulation of ART: The impact of regulation on research and clinical practice. *Journal of Law and Medicine* 9 (May): 399–413.

Jonsen, A.R. 1998. Experiments perilous: The ethics of research with human subjects. In *The Birth of Bioethics,* pp. 125–65. New York: Oxford University Press.

Kaplan, S., and Brownlee, S. 1999. Dying for a cure. *U.S. News and World Report,* October 11.

Kolata, G. 1998. Hope in the lab: A special report. *New York Times,* May 3.

Kolata, G. 2001. Johns Hopkins admits fault in fatal experiment. *New York Times,* July 17.

Kolata, G. 2002. Fertility Inc.: Clinics race to lure clients. *New York Times,* January 1, p. F1.

Korean, G. 2002. Adverse effects of assisted reproductive technology and pregnancy outcome. *Pediatric Research,* 52 (August): 136.

Lambert, R.D. 2002. Safety issues in assisted reproduction technology: The children of assisted reproduction confront the responsible conduct of assisted reproductive technologies. *Human Reproduction* 17 (December): 3011-15.

Levine, R.J. 1979. The boundaries between biomedical or behavioral research and the accepted and routine practice of medicine (July 14, 1974); Addendum (September 24, 1975). In National Commission for the Protection of Human Subjects of Biomedical and Behavioral Research, Boundaries between Research and Practice, Belmont Report, Appendix Volume II, DHEW Publication No. (OS) 78-0014.

Levine, R.J. 1986. *Ethics and Regulations of Clinical Research*, 2nd ed. New Haven: Yale University Press, pp. 3–5.

London, P., and Klerman, G. 1979. Boundaries between research and therapy, especially in mental health. In National Commission for the Protection of Human Subjects of Biomedical and Behavioral Research, Boundaries between Research and Practice, Belmont Report, Appendix Volume II, DHEW Publication No. (OS) 78-0014.

Lorio, K.V. 1999. Symposium: Pushing the boundaries: An interdisciplinary examination of new reproductive technology: The process of regulating assisted reproductive technologies: What we can learn from our neighbors—What translates and what does not. *Loyola Law Review* 45:247–68.

Mack, M., et al. 1999. Inertia of success: A response to minimally invasive coronary bypass: A dissenting opinion. *Circulation* 99:1404–6.

Marcus, A.D. 2002. Key CDC report on fertility clinics is under fire. *Dow Jones Newswires*, December 11.

Margo, C.E. 2001. When is surgery research? Towards an operational definition of human research. *Journal of Medical Ethics* 27:40–43.

Marshall, E. 2000. Gene therapy on trial. *Science* 288:951–57.

McKinlay, J.B. 1981. From "promising report" to "standard procedure": Seven stages in the career of a medical innovation. *Milbank Memorial Fund Quarterly/Health and Society* 59:374–411.

McKneally, M.F., and Daar, A.S. 2003. Introducing new technologies: Protecting subjects of surgical innovation and research. *World Journal of Surgery* 27:930–34.

Miller, G.W. 2000. *King of Hearts: The True Story of the Maverick Who Pioneered Open Heart Surgery.* New York: Three Rivers Press.

Mitchell, A. 2002. Infertility treatment: More risks and challenges (editorial). *New England Journal of Medicine* 346:769–70.

Moore, F.D. 1969. Therapeutic innovation: Ethical boundaries in the initial clinical trials of new drugs and surgical procedures. *Daedalus* (spring).

Moore, F.D. 1988. Three ethical revolutions: Ancient assumptions remodeled under pressure of transplantation. *Transplantation Proceedings* 20 suppl. 1:1061–67.

Moore, F.D. 2000. Ethical problems special to surgery: Surgical teaching, surgical innovation and the surgeon in managed care. *Archives of Surgery* 135:14–16.

Moreno, J.D. 2003. Neuroethics: An agenda for neuroscience and society. *Nature Reviews Neuroscience* 4:149–53.

National Academy of Sciences, National Research Council, Division of Medical Sciences. 1969. *Drug Efficacy Study: Final Report to the Commissioner of Food and Drugs.* Washington, D.C.: National Academy Press.

National Bioethics Advisory Commission. 2001. *Ethical and Policy Issues in Research Involving Human Participants.* Available from www.georgetown.edu/research/nrcb/nbac/pubs.html.

National Institutes of Health, Office of Human Subjects Research, Assurance of Compliance with DHHS Regulations for the Protection of Human Subjects. Available from http://ohsr.od.nih.gov/mpa/mpa.html.

Nelson, D., and Weiss, R. 1999. Hasty decisions in race to a cure? *Washington Post,* November 21.

North, R.L. 2000. Benjamin Rush, MD: beloved healer or assassin? *Baylor University Medical Center Proceedings* 13:45–49.

Ockene, J.K., et al. 2005. Symptom experience after discontinuing use of estrogen plus progestin. *Journal of the American Medical Association* 294:183–93.

O'Toole, K. 1997. The Stanford prison experiment: Still powerful after all these years. *Stanford Report,* January 8. Available from www.stanford.edu/dept/news/pr/97/970108prison exp.html.

Petersen, K. 2002. The regulation of assisted reproductive technology: A comparative study of permissive and prescriptive laws and policies. *Journal of Law and Medicine* 9 (May): 483–97.

Pocock, S.J., et al. 2004. Issues in the reporting of epidemiological studies: A survey of recent practice. *British Medical Journal* 329:883.

Pollack, A. 2003. Hope rises for patient cooling therapy. *New York Times,* August 6, p. 1.

Reitsma, A.M. 2003. Surgical research, an elusive entity. *American Journal of Bioethics* 3:49–50.

Reitsma, A.M., and Moreno, J.D. 2002. Ethical regulations for innovative surgery: The last frontier? *Journal of the American College of Surgery* 194:792–801.

Rennie, D. 1999. Fair conduct and fair reporting of clinical trials. *Journal of the American Medical Association* 282:1766–68.

Robertson, J. 1979. Legal implications of the boundaries between biomedical research involving human subjects and the accepted or routine practice of medicine. In National Commission for the Protection of Human Subjects of Biomedical and Behavioral Research, Boundaries between Research and Practice, Belmont Report, Appendix Volume II, DHEW Publication No. (OS) 78-0014.

Ryan, M. 2002. Countdown to a baby: How hard could it be to get pregnant? *New Yorker,* July 1.

Sabiston, D. 1979. The boundaries between biomedical research involving human subjects and the accepted or routine practice of medicine, with particular emphasis on innovation in the practice of surgery. Page 17-7 in National Commission for the Protection of Human Subjects of Biomedical and Behavioral Research, Boundaries between Research and Practice, Belmont Report, Appendix Volume II, DHEW Publication No. (OS) 78-0014.

Salbu, S.R. 1999. Off-label use, prescription, and marketing of FDA-approved drugs: An assessment of legislation and regulatory policy. *Florida Law Review* 51:181–227.

Serradell, J., and Rucker, T.D. 1990. Prescribing for unlabeled conditions: Patient benefit or therapeutic roulette? *Journal of Pharmaceutical Technology* 6:15–20.

Shaw, D. 2000. Overdose of optimism: A case study in how a story can set off a frenzy. *Los Angeles Times,* February 13, p. A1.

SoRelle, R. 1998. Report on the American Medical Association meeting. *Circulation* 97:516–17.

Spodick, D.H. 1975. Numerators without denominators: There is no FDA for the surgeon. *Journal of the American Medical Association* 232:35–36.

Staudmauer, E.A., et al. 2000. Conventional-dose chemotherapy compared with high-dose chemotherapy plus autologous hematopoietic stem-cell transplantation for metastatic breast cancer. *New England Journal of Medicine* 342:1069–76.

Stelfox, H., et al. 1998. Conflict of interest in the debate over calcium-channel antagonists. *New England Journal of Medicine* 338:101–6.

Stolberg, S.G. 2002. On medicine's frontier: The last journey of James Quinn. *New York Times*, October 8, p. D1.

Tarkan, L. 2002. Fertility clinics begin to address mental health. *New York Times,* October 8, p. D5.

Tulipan, N., Sutton, L.N., Bruner, J.P., et al. 2003. The effect of intrauterine myelomeningocele repair on the incidence of shunt-dependent hydrocephalus. *Pediatric Neurosurgery* 38:27–33.

U.S. Department of Energy, Advisory Committee on Human Radiation Experiments. 1993. Final Report, 1993. Available from www.eh.doe.gov/ohre/roadmap/achre/report.html.

U.S. Department of Health and Human Services, Office for Protection from Research Risks. 2000. Compliance Oversight Investigations Resulting in Restrictions/Actions to Multiple Project Assurances, 1/90–11/99.

U.S. Department of Health and Human Services, Office of Human Research Protections, http://www.hhs.gov/ohrp/.

U.S. Department of Health and Human Services, Office of Inspector General. 1998. Institutional Review Boards: A Time for Reform. June. Available from http://oig.hhs.gov/oei/reports/oei-01-97-00193.pdf.

U.S. General Accounting Office. 1996. Scientific Research: Continued Vigilance Critical to Protecting Human Subjects. March. Available from www.gao.gov/archive/1996/he96072.pdf.

Valenstein, E.S. 1986. *Great and Desperate Cures: The Rise and Decline of Psychosurgery and Other Radical Treatments for Mental Illness.* New York: Basic Books.

Veterans Administration Coronary Artery Bypass Surgery Cooperative Study Group. 1992. Eighteen-year follow-up in the Veterans Affairs Cooperative Study of Coronary Artery Bypass Surgery for stable angina. *Circulation* 86:121–30.

Vollmann, J., and Winau, R. 1996a. Informed consent in human experimentation before the Nuremberg Code. *British Medical Journal* 313:1445–49.

Vollmann, J., and Winau, R. 1996b. The Prussian Regulation of 1900: Early ethical standards for human experimentation in Germany. *IRB: A Review of Human Subject Research* 18:9–11.

Wahlberg, D. 2004. Advertisers probe brains, raise fears. *Atlanta Journal-Constitution,* February 1, p. 1Q.

Wangsness, M. 2000. Pharmacological treatment of obesity: Past, present, and future. *Minnesota Medicine* 83:21–26.

Weiss, R.B. 2001. Breast cancer litigation: Another aspect of the story. *Legal Medicine.* Available from www.afip.org/departments/legalmed/legmed2001/breast.htm.

Weisse, A.B. 2005. Profiles in cardiology: Charles P. Bailey. *Clinical Cardiology* 28: 208–9.

Wells, M. 2003. In search of the buy button. *Forbes,* September 1.

White, C. 2005. Suspected research fraud: Difficulties of getting at the truth. *British Medical Journal* 331:281–88.

Wright, J.M., Lee, C.H., and Chambers, G.K. 1999. Systematic review of antihypertensive therapies: Does the evidence assist in choosing a first-line drug? *Canadian Medical Association Journal* 161:25–32.

Writing Group for the Women's Health Initiative Investigators. 2002. Risks and benefits of estrogen plus progestin in healthy postmenopausal women: Principal results from the Women's Health Initiative Randomized Controlled Trial. *Journal of the American Medical Association* 288:321–33.

Wood, A., Grady, C., and Emanuel, E. 2002. The crisis in human participants research: Identifying the problems and proposing the solutions. Presented to the President's Council on Bioethics, September. Available from http://bioethics.giv/background/emanuelpaper.html.

Zindrick, M.R. 2000. Orthopaedic surgery and Food and Drug Administration off-label uses. *Clinical Orthopaedics and Related Research* 378:31–38.

Index

Margaret L. Eaton, Pharm.D., J.D., received her bachelor's degree in pharmacy from Union University's Albany College of Pharmacy, her doctorate in clinical pharmacy from Duquesne University, and her law degree (cum laude) from the University of California, San Francisco's Hastings College of the Law. She teaches at the Stanford University Graduate School of Business. At the time this book was written, she was a senior research scholar in the Center for Biomedical Ethics at the Stanford University School of Medicine. She has held faculty positions at the University of Minnesota School of Pharmacy and Stanford University. Her non-academic work has included positions at Key Pharmaceuticals, Inc. (clinical research manager), Genentech, Inc. (law clerk), Sedgwick, Detert, Moran & Arnold LLP (litigation attorney in pharmaceutical products liability), and Stanford University (medical attorney in the Office of General Counsel). Dr. Eaton's current teaching includes courses in biotechnology and pharmaceutical business ethics, medical law, and biomedical ethics. Her academic work focuses on the ethical and social issues that affect the biotechnology, pharmaceutical, medical device, and related industries. Among her publications are two books on this subject: *Ethics and the Business of Bioscience* and (with co-authors) *BioIndustry Ethics*.

Donald Kennedy is emeritus Bing Professor of Environmental Science and president emeritus of Stanford University. He received A.B. and Ph.D. degrees in biology from Harvard University and has been on the faculty of Stanford University since 1960. He served as the chairman of the Department of Biology 1964–72 and as director of the then-new Program in Human Biology 1973–77. Dr. Kennedy was commissioner of the U.S. Food and Drug Administration 1977–79 and president of Stanford University 1980–92. He has sat on the National Commission for Public Service and the Carnegie Commission on Science, Technology and Government and is a member of the National Academy of Sciences, the American Academy of Arts and Sciences, and the American Philosophical Society. Currently he co-chairs the NAS Project on Science, Technology and Law. Since June 2000 he has been editor-in-chief of *Science*, the journal of the American Association for the Advancement of Science. Dr. Kennedy's present research, conducted through the Institute for International Studies at Stanford, consists of interdisciplinary studies on the development of policies regarding such transboundary environmental problems as major land-use changes, economically driven alterations in agricultural practice, and global climate change.